start talking

start
talking

A Girl's Guide for You and Your Mom about Health, Sex, or Whatever

[an inside look at the details
even *she* doesn't know!]

mary jo rapini &
janine sherman

Bayou
Publishing
HOUSTON, TX

This publication is designed to provide accurate and authoritative information in regard to the subject matter covered. It is sold with the understanding that the publisher is not engaged in rendering legal, accounting, psychotherapeutic or other professional service. If expert assistance is required, the services of a competent professional person should be sought. From a Declaration of Principles jointly adopted by a Committee of the American Bar Association and a Committee of Publishers.

Editing: Steve Sherman, Bety Jo Caid, Jennifer Schaffer
Back Cover Copywritng: Susan Kendrick—Susan Kendrick Writing
Cover Design: Kathi Dunn—Dunn & Associates
Cover Illustration: Buffy Espersen
Illustrations: Cynthia Burtch— Pro Tech Studio
Printing: United Graphics, Inc.

Printed in the United States of America
First Edition 10 9 8 7 6 5 4 3 2 1

Publisher's Cataloging-in-Publication
(Provided by Quality Books, Inc.)

Rapini, Mary Jo.
    Start talking : a girl's guide for you and your mom
about health, sex, or whatever / Mary Jo Rapini, Janine
Sherman. -- 1st ed.
    p. cm. -- (Talk at the table series ; 1)
    Includes bibliographical references and index.
    LCCN 2008925866
    ISBN-13: 978-1-886298-31-6
    ISBN-10: 1-886298-31-9

    1. Teenage girls--Health and hygiene. 2. Sex
instruction for girls. 3. Mothers and daughters.
4. Comunication in the family.   I. Sherman, Janine.
II. Title. III. Title: Girl's guide for you and your mom
about health, sex, or whatever. IV. Series.

RA777.25.R37 2008   613'.04243
                    QBI08-600129

Published by Bayou Publishing
2524 Nottingham • Houston, TX 77005-1412
713-526-4558 • http://www.bayoupublishing.com

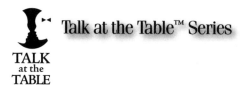

TALK
at the
TABLE

Talk at the Table™ Series

CONTENTS

NOTE TO THE READER

This book is a joint project—the outgrowth of our talks together, consultations together, presentations to women's health providers, shared frustrations, joint visions. We each have stories to contribute. We both have definite opinions, yet we have not distinguished between our contributions to this book. At times "I" refers to Mary Jo, and other times to Janine, but could very well be either of us. We have chosen to share our stories and answer questions without specifically identifying who is talking. Please join us as we talk around the table.

INTRODUCTION

T eens today, more than ever, face a myriad of issues involving sex and sexuality, self-esteem and body image. They need education; they need guidance; they need support to make the right decisions at the right time.

In our profession as women's health care providers, we've found that teens experience greater success through these difficult years when they have open communication with their mothers.

But we've also found that's not quite as simple as it sounds.

As women's health care providers we understand that daughters are commonly reluctant to approach their mothers for advice, for fear of punishment or lecture, or simply because they are embarrassed of the issue itself. They instead turn to their friends or the mass media, or avoid the issues all together, creating greater problems for themselves in the future.

And as mothers ourselves, we also understand that many of us are embarrassed to admit that despite our best intentions, we hesitate to engage our daughters in health-related dialogue. We either feel shy, inadequate, and poorly informed, or we have been so looking forward to such interactions with our daughters—anticipating with cherished thoughts how our conversations will go, only to discover that our teenage daughters are disinterested, busy, or outright offended.

So where are teen girls getting the little information they do have about health and sex? And what is it that they are concluding about health and sex and their bodies from these information sources? Adolescent girls learn about sex primarily from their conversations with their *mothers*, interactions with their *peers*, participation in *school programs*, and exposure to *mass media*, yet not necessarily in that order. All contribute to the knowledge our children receive about sex and their bodies; all are potential sources of conversation with our daughters.

Mothers. As mothers, from the time that our children are born, we make sure that they are clean, fed and clothed. We take them to the pediatrician regularly. We teach them everything, from how to ride a bike to how to use appropriate manners. We provide our children with love, protection and guidance. We tend to breeze through most of these tasks, and when we stumble occasionally, we turn to our own mothers for help.

As our children become more inquisitive and their lives become more complicated, these tasks can become far more challenging. Most of us find it uncomfortable when our daughters ask us questions about sex and their bodies. We often have difficulty teaching our daughters about sex because of our own discomfort and/or our own lack of knowledge. This uneasiness with the subject is often a reflection of the way that we were taught about sex by our own mothers, years earlier.

> My mother had only two significant conversations with me about my body and sex, which were probably two more conversations than she had with her own mother. Our first conversation was about menstruation, and we had it just before I actually started getting my periods. Oversimplified and incomplete, the information that she provided was probably all she felt was needed to handle my first episode of bleeding.

> Our second conversation, when I was 13 years old, was about human reproduction. My mother read me a book, which had been recommended by her gynecologist, entitled "How to Talk to 6-8 Year Olds." Like other mothers, she was uncomfortable about teaching me what I needed to know about sex and my body. Also, like other mothers, her knowledge about sexuality and related

*health issues may have been limited. Our conversations were a
beginning but they did not provide me with all the information that
I would need as a teen.*

Peers. Adolescent girls exert a huge influence on each other. This is a time in a girl's life when she desperately wants to "fit in." Peers help each other "figure it all out." Teen girls can also be a fabulous resource for *inaccurate* information.

Young girls also get a lot of inaccurate information from their boyfriends — whom they want to please — about the risks of sexual activity. For example, a common myth believed by boys is that girls can't get pregnant "the first time."

Never underestimate the influence girls have on each other regarding the issue of body image. It's been noted, for instance, that eating disorders can "run in packs." Girls teach each other how to "do it" and encourage each other to stay skinny. The concern to "be popular" or "fit in" is far more important than taking care of their bodies. They find out what it means to be *popular* and to *fit in*, first and foremost from their buddies.

School Programs. Our public schools are another primary source of sex education for girls. In 1996, the federal government enacted legislation limiting federal funding for sex education programs in public school to those programs with an "abstinence only" curriculum. Those programs focus on sex after marriage, ignore pre-marital sex, and do not mention birth control and safe sex practices. As parents, abstinence until marriage sounds like a great idea for our daughters. Unfortunately, as a public policy, it has not proven particularly effective.

A recent public health study not only confirms that teen girls generally are not abstaining from sexual intercourse, but demonstrates that 75% of females have had premarital sex by the age of 20. Further, by not emphasizing the need for safe sex practices if a girl decides not to abstain, school-based programs fail to show our girls how to protect their health. Fewer than 10% of sexually active teenagers are using condoms when having sex. Consequently, adolescents have the highest prevalence of sexually transmitted diseases.

Teenagers are surging with natural hormonal urges, yet they are not being taught in school how to deal with them. This is like putting hungry children in a room with all kinds of food. Most of them would take the junk food instead of the healthier alternatives unless we have taught them how to make better choices.

Mass media. The fourth, and perhaps the most influential source of information about sex is the mass media. From magazines to television to the Internet to radio—from every source you can think of—the message is the same. Each source screams "SEX" at adolescents. Prime time network television shows an average of eight sexual incidents per hour. Almost half of adolescents report learning about sex, pregnancy, and birth control from television, movies and magazines. Movies and television are powerful educators, often portraying reckless and unsafe behavior by teens in a glamorous or romantic light. Sex, as portrayed by the media, frequently involves quick hook-ups and immediate gratification.

Even in the absence of frank references to sex, magazines and other media targeting adolescent girls emphasize "ideal" body images and suggestive behaviors to attract boys sexually. As a result, girls are encouraged to have unhealthy diets and engage in practices with sex as the ultimate goal. For instance, look at any teen oriented fashion magazine; all of the models are unrealistically thin and the articles range from "how to kiss better" to "how to get *him* to notice you."

Health care providers often see young women *after* problems occur— problems that might have been avoided if the adolescents had received adequate education, or if they had found opportunities to engage a *trusted, meaningful person* with their questions. When we mothers fall short in educating our girls about health, sex, and self-esteem we miss out on our opportunities to prevent potential problems. We cannot count on the schools, our daughters' peers or the mass media to provide our adolescent daughters with the information that they need to protect themselves.

The goal of this book is to empower mothers and daughters with accurate and comprehensive knowledge so that they can have the open, relaxed, and informative conversations about sex and female health that every young woman needs and deserves. Mothers have the chance to directly shape their daughters' thought processes regarding their bodies, life choices, health and well being. The book also highlights the mother-daughter connection in helping girls to explore their passions and to focus their energies on self discovery.

For you mothers, *table talk* is a way of comfortably inviting your daughter into your beliefs and thoughts, and learning from her as well. For you daughters, *table talk* is a way of comfortably inviting your mother into your beliefs and thoughts, and learning from her as well. *This book is designed for both moms and daughters alike.* The information is meant to be shared. It is deliberately meant to spark conversations. Getting started with *table talk* can happen almost any place or time, just as this book describes.

Young girls deserve accurate information presented in a relaxed way by people whom they trust. They deserve straightforward answers to their questions. Moms deserve a chance to have engaging conversations with their daughters about life-critical issues.

TABLE TALK

Setting the Table. Here are great mother-daughter ideas for "settings" to have table talk conversations:

• Ride with just the two of you in the car listening to music. The lyrics can often spur great conversations.

• Take a walk—a wandering walk—together, and let the conversation go where it may.

• Pick your daughter up from school and suggest a drink at a coffee house. Most coffee houses have comfortable seating and generally are quiet at this time of day.

• Go to a knitting shop and learn to knit together. Many such shops often have quiet, cozy areas in which to work. Furthermore, knitting can be a productive conversation-enhancing hobby.

• Read a book together, followed by discussion sessions. Let the book's content be your conversation starters.

- *Make plans to get up early and have a quiet breakfast before the rest of the family wakes up.*

- *Go to yoga class together and get a smoothie afterwards. Yoga puts everyone in a good mood.*

- *Dance together. Enroll in a tap class, then have dinner afterwards.*

- *Plant an herb garden and cook one meal per week together.*

- *Have a "spa day" at home. Buy a facial mask and give each other "manis" and "pedis." Serve sparkling apple cider to make it seem really special.*

- *One afternoon find a place in your town that has high tea. If unable to find a place with high tea, make scones, put on classical music and have a tea party.*

- *On a sunny day make a picnic lunch and go to a local park.*

- *Find a pottery painting place and do some artwork.*

- *Try working out together. It can make exercising more fun!*

Getting started with *table talk* can happen almost any place or any time. Putting the facts on the table and learning from one another may be the best gift a mother can give her daughter to protect her future health.

> *My favorite way to talk to my daughter at night is when she gets on her treadmill at her school gym and I get on mine at home. We put our phones on speaker and talk to each other as we walk. It's like being on a walk together even when we are miles apart. It also makes exercise more fun, and I am connected with her throughout my dreams at night.*

CHAPTER 1

"Oops ... I Had an Accident"

UNDERSTANDING MENSTRUATION

*M*ost girls in the fourth or fifth grade now bring home a note from school, requesting permission to watch a film on menstruation. At my girls' public elementary school, the parents are given the option to preview the film or to attend the viewing of the film with their daughters. Each child must have a permission slip signed by a parent allowing her to view the movie. I am told that few parents actually go to preview the film.

I figured that I didn't need to preview the film because my girls had long been familiar with tampons, sanitary pads, and the other accompaniments of menstruation. Furthermore, I planned to be at the actual showing. When the inevitable question "what *are these for" was asked by one of the girls holding a pad in her hand (or, in the case of one daughter, on her head), the question was answered honestly and in a straightforward manner. My oldest daughter was happy to have me come to her class, but much to my surprise, there was only one other mother in attendance at the viewing of the film.*

When I mentioned to the other fourth grade moms that I had seen the film with my daughter, most of them told me that they didn't want to make their daughter feel uncomfortable by being there themselves. I wondered what might be so uncomfortable about discussing menstruation, knowing that all healthy women eventually have periods and have to deal with menses for many years, and at this point, I reminisced back to my childhood.

When I was an adolescent, I had first learned about my period through one of my friends at school who proceeded to show me the "diapers" we would have to wear when we started bleeding from "down there." After that horrifying experience, I went home in search of the "diapers" because I was sure this friend had to be lying to me. Sure enough, there they were in my sister's and mom's bathrooms. I concluded that this must be something we didn't talk about, because who would want to tell her daughter that she would bleed and have to wear a diaper! I had so many questions: Did you bleed forever? When would this start? These and other questions entered my mind, with no answers in sight.

My goal was to get my sister or mom to verify this story without me having to ask them directly. I first tried to see if my sister would tell me, so I went into the bathroom while she was putting on make-up, reached into the cabinet under the sink, grabbed the box of sanitary napkins, and pretended to drop them accidentally. Instead of recognizing this as an opportunity to educate her younger sister, she very nonchalantly returned the napkins to the cabinet and banished me from the bathroom.

The next attempt I made to obtain reliable information about bleeding and those mysterious diapers came when my mother and I were strolling down the grocery store aisle that contained the feminine hygiene products. I planned to ask casually what they were and why people bought them. As we approached them, I was working out in my head exactly what I would say to my mother that would not make either one of us uncomfortable. At the last moment, when we were right in front of the boxes of sanitary napkins, I "chickened out."

My quest continued for several months. Finally, one day when I had stayed home from school because I had a stomach ache, I was helping my mom in the kitchen. She casually asked me if there was anything messy or unusual in my panties. I had no idea what she meant or exactly what she was going to say, so I firmly replied "NO!" She proceeded to tell me that one day I might see blood in my panties, that this would be normal, and that I should just come and let her know. That was the full extent of our first conversation about menstrual periods.

Sure enough, I woke up early one morning, and there it was: Blood. I ran in to my parents' room and woke my mom up. She gave me sanitary napkins and a belt to hold the pad in place, and after some basic instructions, she sent me on my way. I definitely did not feel like celebrating this mark of womanhood, and I certainly did not think that this was a good day. At school, I really felt like I was wearing a diaper, and I was terrified that somehow everyone would know that I got my period. I later discovered that I was one of the very first of my peers to have a period. I viewed it as a curse.

Every month I came to dread the approach of my menses. My mom would casually ask me how I was, and my pat answer was always that I was "fine." From my perspective, I certainly didn't feel that we could suddenly start comfortably discussing menstruation after having avoided the topic for so long. Looking back, my mom probably felt that she had made huge strides in communication compared with her mom, who I later found had talked even less to my mom about her impending period.

Eventually, at my Catholic school, it came time to watch "the film." By this point, I felt that I was a pro, but I still didn't want other people to know I had started having periods. Along with the rest of the girls, I laughed and paid little attention to the actual facts contained in the movie, while the nuns sat in class with us.

At the viewing of the film in my daughter's school, I realized that not much had changed since my childhood. There was a lot of giggling, and many of the girls were ignoring the film completely. The teacher referred many of the girls' questions to me as a women's health professional, worsening my daughter's humiliation of having one of the only two mothers who attended the viewing. Several years later, when my younger daughter had to go through this process, she simply requested that I not come to the school.

Needless to say, when each of my daughters started having menstrual cycles, they understood what was happening. They believed themselves to be completely prepared for it. We had talked about this for so long and in such a matter-of-fact manner that they were, unlike myself at their age, quite relieved to start their periods!

The menstrual cycle discussion is often the first conversation a mother and daughter will have that directly relates to women's health or female sexuality. It is not uncommon, however, for a mother to be uncomfortable when this discussion arises, relying instead on school curricula or the media to teach her daughter.

To get started on this conversation about menstruation with your daughter, it's important to know the facts, the clinical aspects behind this monthly inconvenience. It's also important to use simple, easy-to-understand language in describing the basic facts.

Any *table talk conversation* about menstruation will stall if it gets bogged down in a compendium of medical reports. Take advantage of opportunities that present themselves; for instance, if your daughter asks about sanitary napkins, frankly but in a relaxed tone answer the questions. Remember, children have great radar, so the more comfortable you are when you answer questions the more relaxed they will be.

WELCOME TO MENSTRUATION 101

Starting your cycle is a sign that your reproductive system is maturing. Most of us moms had to sit through boring, stiff films at about 8-10 years of age to learn about our cycles. Most of us, admittedly, were too embarrassed to pay attention and came out with little more understanding of our cycle than when the film started. Since most moms themselves don't understand this process, they have a difficult time explaining it to their daughters. Indeed, many women have no desire to learn more as long as their periods are normal.

However, a basic understanding of the menstrual cycle can put you in touch with certain symptoms that will be experienced throughout the month. Remember: *knowledge is empowering. It makes conversations easier.*

The three main body parts that are basic to menstruation are the *pituitary gland*, the *ovaries*, and the *uterus*.

Now the pathway between the pituitary gland and the ovaries is a very delicate one. (Ovaries are where eggs are made.) Think of this pathway as a road that hormones travel. The pituitary gland sits at the base of the brain and sends hormones to the ovaries, instructing the glands to produce other hormones for ovulation. Hormones are messengers that trigger the events of your cycle, but to many young girls the immaturity of this pathway can be the cause of most menstrual problems. The term ovulation refers to the release of a mature egg.

The ovaries are in the pelvis and are responsible for the production of women's sex hormones in the body. They in turn send signals back to the pituitary about hormone levels that are being produced by the ovaries. It may be easier to think of it like a household thermostat. The pituitary tells the ovaries to start working, much like a thermostat tells the heater to start working as it registers a drop in temperature. When the pituitary starts sending too strong a message, though, the ovaries tell it to back off.

The uterus is where a fetus grows. The lining of the uterus is determined by the hormones produced by the ovaries. These hormones are *estrogen, progesterone*, and *testosterone*. (Yes, testosterone is not just for boys. Girls have testosterone, too. Don't worry; it's not enough testosterone to grow a beard.) Estrogen is the most prominent sex hormone in your body. From about day one to day 14, the pituitary is sending the message to your ovaries to produce estrogen and to start developing follicles, which are immature eggs in the ovaries. Even though you have two ovaries, only one works at a time.

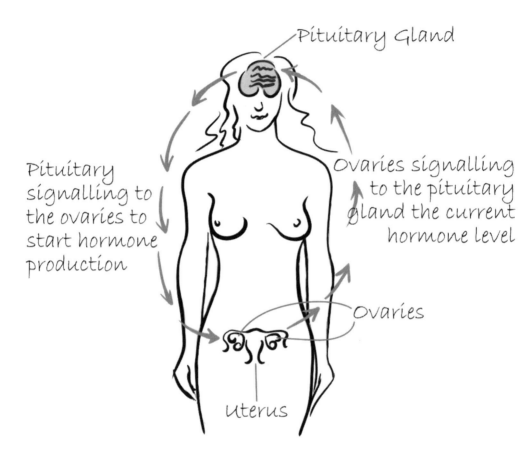

Pituitary Gland

Pituitary signalling to the ovaries to start hormone production

Ovaries signalling to the pituitary gland the current hormone level

Ovaries

Uterus

During this time of the month, the higher levels of estrogen send signals to the uterine lining to thicken up in case it has to support the needs of a fertilized egg for nine months.

Around the time of ovulation, which occurs at mid-cycle, testosterone levels go up, and the body begins to naturally hunt for sperm. Often, girls have a higher sex drive around mid-cycle because testosterone levels go up. When the egg matures enough to be ovulated, it leaves the ovary and travels down the fallopian tube toward the uterus in search of fertilization. The egg is only able to be fertilized for about 24-48 hours after ovulation. After the egg leaves the ovary, the corpus luteum, a small fluid filled area, is left behind. The corpus luteum starts

Uterine Changes During Menstrual Cycle

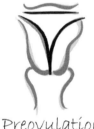 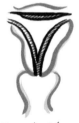 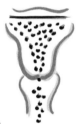

Preovulation
(with thin lining)

Ovulation
(Thickening of the
lining after ovulation)

Starting your period
(Breaking down of
the uterine lining)

producing progesterone, which will help the uterus to maintain the early pregnancy *just in case* the egg is fertilized.

During the second half of the cycle, or days 14-28, progesterone is the main hormone produced by the ovary. The message is sent to the lining of the uterus to start maturing. If pregnancy does not occur, then the message that the pituitary sends to the ovaries is for the sex hormones to begin to fall. This fall in sex hormones, especially progesterone, causes the inner lining of the uterus to begin to fall apart, which starts the bleeding process we call "the period." When the bleeding stops, the pituitary starts again to send the message to the ovaries to make female sex hormones, and the entire cycle starts all over again.

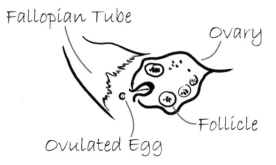

There you have it. We know all of this information can seem a little confusing and (let's be honest) perhaps a little boring. Growing up means learning more about your body and how it functions. It is important to know what's going on, so you can also tell when something is going wrong.

Now, enough technical stuff on periods; it's Q&A time. Let's have some girl talk about periods.

DAUGHTER QUESTIONS

Girls, daughters, we just presented some things for you to know about your menstrual cycles *from a clinical standpoint*. Here are typical questions that girls often ask when they visit the OB-GYN (obstetrician/ gynecologist) or other health care provider. Think about any other questions you might have beyond what's listed here. Remember that for answers to those questions a great resource is your mom. She's been down this road as well.

Q: What is the normal age a girl gets her period? When can I expect it to happen to me?

A: Well, a girl's first period, called *menarche*, can start as early as eight or as late as 16 years old. And though the average age is 11, starting your period later in life is *not necessarily abnormal.* Now with that being said, if you are 15 with no signs that you've begun hormone production (breasts beginning to develop, hair growth under the arms and in the pubic area), you need to see a health care provider. If you still haven't begun your period by the time you're 16, no matter where you are developmentally, you need to see a health care provider.

Q: But how do I know it's near?

A: Look for other signs and symptoms that your first cycle is near. These include acne or breaking out of the skin, mood changes, growth spurts, and the need for use of underarm deodorants. Also, you may begin to notice small amounts of discharge in your panties. When you notice these changes, it is a good time to talk to your mom about buying pads to have on hand in case you start your period.

TABLE TALK

Conversations about Body Change. Don't start the conversation if either party is stressed out or you don't have time to talk. Start by bringing up the fact that your body is changing. In this particular case you start out by requesting the need for a bra.

Miranda (daughter): Mom, my friend just got her first bra and I think it's time for me to start wearing a bra.

Abigail (Mom): You know I was starting to notice that your body was changing. We can go on a shopping expedition to buy some bras. Have you noticed any other changes?

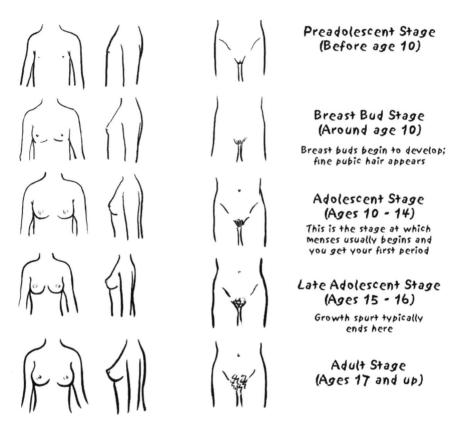

Preadolescent Stage
(Before age 10)

Breast Bud Stage
(Around age 10)

Breast buds begin to develop;
fine pubic hair appears

Adolescent Stage
(Ages 10 - 14)

This is the stage at which
menses usually begins and
you get your first period

Late Adolescent Stage
(Ages 15 - 16)

Growth spurt typically
ends here

Adult Stage
(Ages 17 and up)

Tanner Stages of
Body Development Across the Life Span

Miranda: My gym coach tells me I need to wear deodorant more regularly and I am getting hair in places I didn't have it before.

Abigail: It happens to all growing girls. Do you have any concerns or questions about these changes?

Miranda: The question I have is how soon do you think I will get my period?

Abigail: There's no way of knowing for sure "when," but the more your body matures the closer your period is.

Q: Should I worry if my periods are not the same each month? Does that make me weird or abnormal?

A: It is common when you first start your period to have irregular cycles. That's OK. We sometimes call them *abnormal cycles*, mainly because feedback from your pituitary to your ovaries doesn't work well when you are having your first cycles, but it will eventually become more regular as time goes on.

Long cycles are cycles that last longer than one week. Again, it is usually the poor communication between the pituitary gland and the ovaries that is the cause of long cycles. If you consistently bleed longer than a week you should see your health care provider.

Cycles can come as often as 22 days or as far apart as 35 days and still be considered normal. It is not uncommon for young girls to skip several months when they first start their periods, but if after three months you still haven't gotten your next period, you should consult a health care provider. A cycle that comes more frequently than every three weeks on a consistent basis is also considered to be abnormal.

But if you are having sex, you should see a health care provider as soon as you realize you have skipped your period. It is important to *make sure you are not pregnant.*

Q: What about really heavy cycles?

A: *Heavy cycles* are usually associated with hormone imbalances due to immaturity of the menstrual cycle. A cycle is too heavy if you have to change your pad more than every couple of hours. I have had young girls come to my office because they could not get through a class period without bleeding through their pad. If this is a common occurrence, you need to see a women's health care provider.

Most of these abnormal issues can be taken care of. The most important lesson here is *if your period is abnormal, don't freak out.* It can usually be fixed fairly easily, without even taking your clothes off. It's up to you, though, to talk to someone and get an appointment with a health care provider.

Q: I get a headache before I start my period each month. Why does this happen?

A: Headaches that occur with your cycle are called *menstrual migraines*, and are caused by blood vessels expanding in the brain. They often occur a few days before you start bleeding and are severe in nature, lasting from several hours to several days. These headaches are thought to go along with the hormonal drops that occur to make your period start.

Some birth control pills are designed specifically to help with menstrual migraines by adding small amounts of estrogen to the *sugar pills*, which are the last week of the pack. The estrogen prevents the big drop in hormones thought to trigger the headache. These pills work quite well, but if you don't want to use oral contraceptives, using migraine headache medication can also work well. (For more detail on how birth control pills work, see pages 121-123).

Q: Why do you cramp while you're on your period?

A: Severe cramps are defined as *painful periods*. The medical term is *dysmenorrhea*. There are certain factors that put people at risk for having cramps, such as being under the age of 20, experiencing heavy periods, smoking (just another good reason not to smoke!), depression, anxiety, stress, poor diet, as well as not ever having been pregnant.

Q: Really? Getting pregnant reduces cramps?

A: Typically, but this is not a reason to go get pregnant. Trust me on that one! Cramps are the most common reason why girls are absent from school and work. Some studies show that up to 90% of women get cramps during adolescence.

There are many reasons why you get cramps. The most important two reasons are *prostaglandins* and *ischemia*. Prostaglandins are strong, hormone-like substances released into the menstrual fluid that cause uterine muscles to contract, causing pain. This contracting is also believed to produce a decrease in oxygen flowing to the muscles of the uterus, or ischemia, which also increases the pain and cramping. Sometimes painful periods are a sign of early endometriosis.

Lindsay, a 13 year old girl in 8th grade, and her mother came into the office because of heavy bleeding from her period. For the past two days since her period had begun, she was having to change her sanitary napkin every 45-60 minutes to prevent bleeding through to her clothes. Her very first period came about five months prior and although the periods came every 4-6 weeks they were getting heavier each month. This most recent cycle was the worst. The period was not slowing down at all and Lindsay was complaining about feeling light-headed when she stood up. Lindsay was normal weight and had normal physical development.

The goal of the visit was to stop the bleeding, or at least to make it more manageable. The best way to do this is with birth control pills. Lindsay was given a sample pack of pills and instructed to begin taking them that day. Because she had become anemic (i.e., dangerously low on iron from loss of blood), she was also given iron tablets to help raise her blood count.

In addition, she was instructed to come back in a few weeks for follow-up, unless the bleeding did not slow down within a few days, in which case she was to immediately call the office. When she returned to the office, her bleeding had stopped within two days of starting the medication, and the iron in her blood count was within the normal range.

The big question became whether to keep her on the pill and for how long. She (and her mother) wanted to know how long she would have to continue taking the pill. Together, we came to the decision to continue the pill for two more months, allowing her blood count to stay stable. We would then discontinue and reevaluate her cycles. Within three months after she stopped taking birth control pills, her periods came at four week intervals. Better yet, they were significantly lighter. This was probably due to the normal maturation that occurs in the body over time.

Q: I hear people tease my sister about PMS. What is PMS?

A: My house has three menstruating girls, so I often refer to it as a hotbed for *premenstrual syndrome* or PMS. No one fully understands why we get PMS, but it is believed that it is related to hormonal fluctuations that occur after ovulation and before you start you period. (Remember when we talked about that in "Welcome to Menstrual 101"?) The symptoms can be physical, emotional or behavioral.

It is thought that 60-80% of women have PMS. PMS occurs on average 2-14 days prior to the onset of your period and leaves 24-48 hours after you start bleeding. If you think you have symptoms every day of your cycle, it is not PMS. Some of the symptoms include: breast tenderness, general bloating, headaches, fatigue, food cravings, moodiness, anxiety, tearfulness, and depression. Symptoms can range from mild to severe.

Q: Can I do anything about PMS ... you know, hide it even?

A: Some simple things you can try to curtail symptoms of PMS are to eat properly, which also means limiting caffeine, sugar and salt. In other words, watch the colas and chips. Exercise regularly. Get plenty of sleep. Supplements that help with PMS that I like to recommend are Calcium 1200mg/ day (especially important if you don't get it in your diet), and Magnesium 400 mg/day. Both of these have shown to decrease PMS symptoms. Vitamin B6 has been shown to have limited use but is thought to act as a natural diuretic (encourages urination), so it may help with breast tenderness and bloating. Chaste berry fruit at 20 mg/day has been shown to help with moodiness.

If symptoms are more than mild and frequently interfere with your daily life, you should visit your health care provider to discuss birth control pills. The pill is often very helpful for premenstrual symptoms. Additionally, some antidepressants are very effective for mood problems associated with PMS.

Q: At what age is it safe for me to start wearing tampons?

A: That all depends on how comfortable you are using them. Tampons are a method of menstrual protection that has been around for over 60 years. They are those absorbent, cotton sticks that are inserted into the vagina with a cardboard or plastic applicator, and a cotton string that hangs out of the vagina for easy removal. Some young girls find that sanitary napkins (pads) aren't comfortable or they get in the way of certain activities such as swimming, and are anxious to start wearing tampons. Other girls are in no rush to insert anything into their vaginas, and that is fine.

The best way to start using tampons is to start with the smallest, most slender tampons available on the market. The instructions inside the package will show you positions that help the vaginal muscles to relax. (A water-based lubricant like K-Y Jelly® can be used to help as well). If you are too nervous to insert them, there is no rush. However, if you think the vaginal opening isn't big enough (which means you cannot insert a finger), see your health care provider. *Remember, your vagina does not bite.*

Q: How often should I change my tampons? Can I sleep in them?

A: The most important thing about wearing tampons is remembering to change them often. There is an infection called Toxic Shock Syndrome (TSS) that has rarely been associated with tampon use. TSS can be deadly if not caught in time, but it can certainly be prevented by not leaving a tampon in too long. TSS comes from a certain type of bacteria that can rapidly grow in a closed space, and wearing a tampon too long can facilitate the growth of the bacteria. *Therefore, tampons are safe if you CHANGE them regularly.* I recommend changing them every 4-6 hours and not sleeping in them.

Q: What should I do if I think I have left a tampon in and can't find it?

A: About once a month a patient comes in and tells us that she thinks she has left a tampon in her vagina and cannot find it. About half the time we find a tampon and about half the time we do not. The message is that if you think there is any possibility that you have left one in, go see your health care provider and make sure. Don't be embarrassed if there is not one. It is better to be safe than sorry. On the other hand, people come in for routine check ups, saying that they have a funny odor. Lo and behold! When we examine them, there's a tampon in the vagina!

If you have further questions, talk to your mother and see what she suggests. Try it; you may be surprised to find you're not as embarrassed as you think you will be talking to her. In fact, read on for some good questions you could ask your mother.

Q: What do I do about really bad cramps?

A: If you feel like your uterus is being tied in knots, there are certain measures you can take to ease the pain. Sometimes, simple over-the-counter treatments or diet changes can be enough to ward off the pain. For a number of girls, though, it can take prescription medicines or daily vitamins to solve the problems. My first word of advice is to try taking non-steroidal, anti-inflammatory drugs like ibuprofen. Medicines like ibuprofen directly decrease prostaglandin release.

It is important to treat your pain as soon as you notice it. For instance, if it is time for your period and you notice some cramping, go ahead and take the medicine. Don't wait until the pain is so bad you can't move! It is much harder to stop severe pain than it is to prevent it if you treat it at a milder stage.

If you take medicines like ibuprofen once a month for a day or two and you have no reactions to ibuprofen, just plan on doing it regularly. Take it before the pain interferes with your life. This is one of the most effective treatments since it works directly on the cause of the cramping. This is also the simplest treatment since you can buy it inexpensively anywhere, and you don't need a prescription.

Q: I don't like taking those pain pills. Is there anything else I can do?

A: Another way to manage severe cramps is birth control pills. Oral contraceptives treat menstrual cramps very successfully by decreasing flow and prostaglandin release. The downside to this method is that you have to go to your health care provider for a prescription, and you must remember to take them every day.

A low-fat, vegetarian diet and exercise are two examples of lifestyle changes that have been shown to help cramps. If you are looking for a reason to give up meat, this could be one. Whether you give up meat or not, however, a balanced, healthy diet is important to all facets of life. Exercise has been shown to be beneficial also, because it can lead to increased blood flow to the uterus. In my opinion, regular exercise is good all around because it leads to release of endorphins in the brain, which are natural pain relievers and will make you feel better! I am a particular fan of Pilates and yoga because they also exercise your mind and spirit.

Q: Is there something "natural" I can do?

A: Other, more natural and alternative treatments are occasionally used for the treatment of cramps. Thiamine, at a dosage of 100mg/day, has shown in some cultures to be successful. In the U.S., however, the typical diet is not low in thiamine (which is a B vitamin), and this supplement probably isn't necessary or helpful here. Vitamin E, taken at 2,500 IU for five days, starting two days prior to your period, has been shown to decrease pain. This is a large dose, so I don't encourage this one very often, but there is research that supports its use. Fish oil at 2 gm/day has been shown to have some benefits in treating pain associated with periods. Fish oil has many other health benefits, so I would encourage this treatment most often.

There are other less common treatments like acupuncture and Chinese herbal medicines that have shown some success for treating menstrual cramps. Although there is some scientific evidence that these treatments will work, they may not be widely available.

And don't forget about that good ol' heating pad. Sometimes, just cuddling up with a heating pad is enough to get you feeling back to normal. Remember not to fall asleep with it or to let it get too hot.

You can always ask your mom what she does for cramps. My daughters and I often find ourselves **swapping period tips and stories**. But remember that everyone's body works differently, and what works for your friend or sister may not work for you. Talk to your mother; ask her for recommendations. She's been dealing with this issue for years.

Q: Talking about this period stuff is embarrassing, especially around my dad or brother. How can I talk about it in a way I won't get embarrassed?

A: Hopefully, your dad is somewhat comfortable with periods since he probably has had some experience from your mom with menstruation. If you notice that he is uncomfortable about the subject, mention it to him, because he may not be aware of the vibes he is sending out. As far as your brother goes, it can actually be very good for your brother to become comfortable with the topic, since he may one day be involved with a woman. Having some basic knowledge about cycles can make him more understanding about her cycles. The more comfortable you are talking about the subject, the more relaxed they will be hearing about it.

MOM QUESTIONS

Moms, let's take a look at some of your questions about menstruation. Here are some frequently encountered ones to get you started on having open conversations with your daughters about her period.

Q: What are signs that my daughter is about to start her menstrual cycle?

A: Female development is a slow process. In general the physical changes begin around age 10. Often the first sign that your daughter's body is starting to mature is the need for underarm deodorant. Body odor is the sign that hormone production is starting to occur. The next most common sign is the development of breast buds, a little bit of tissue under the nipples. The adolescent growth spurt begins. Around a year later the sparse growth of pubic hair will begin. The process from the onset of signs of maturing to the onset of menstruation is about two years.

Q: What steps should I take to prepare my daughter for her menstrual cycle?

A: As your daughter's body begins to mature, it is time to prepare your daughter for her cycle with equipment (e.g., purchasing tampons or sanitary pads). Buy and talk; talk and buy.

When my oldest daughter went to sleep-away camp in seventh grade she was certainly developing. When we arrived at camp I marched her to the nurse's office and explained to the nurse that my daughter could start her period while at camp and she was fully equipped. The nurse kind of chuckled but reassured me and sent me on my way. Two days prior to picking her up from camp, I received a letter from my daughter. She informed me that she had gone horseback riding, swam in the lake, and, oh, by the way, got her period.

With no quick way to contact her, you can imagine my anticipation to see if she was all right. When I arrived to pick her up, it became clear to me that she felt that getting her period was just another day in her life. During that same time, a number of the girls in her cabin also started their cycles and she helped them out. Even though I personally felt left out when I received the letter, I was very pleased that she was so well prepared, and proud that she reached out to help others.

Q: My daughter is 14. She got her first period eight months ago and she has only had 4 cycles, all of which seemed very heavy. Should I take her to the doctor?

A: First of all, it is very common for girls to have irregular cycles when they first get their period. The message sent by the pituitary to the ovaries often doesn't work smoothly when girls first start their periods and the result is irregular cycles. If she is saturating a sanitary pad in less than two hours, that is too heavy and she would need to seek medical care.

The problem with periods that are heavy is the risk of becoming anemic from losing too much blood. Often in this case, I will put a patient on birth control pills to control her bleeding and to allow her blood count to rebound to normal. Supplemental iron is often recommended to help make new red blood cells.

Q: When is the best time to begin talking to my daughter about her cycle?

A: The best time to talk to your daughter is as soon as she makes any inquiry about it. My oldest daughter started asking me about sanitary napkins at about age five; I was extremely basic yet honest in my answer. I told her that when she got older she would have a cycle each month and that the napkins were for that. I am certain it did not fully sink into her head what that meant. However, the answer was honest and factual.

Kids sense when you are uncomfortable discussing something, or when you are avoiding the topic or not being honest. Think of it like this: no one is afraid to tell their child that one day they will know how to ride a bike, which is a developmental milestone. The same should hold true when it comes to your daughter's period. Remind your daughter that getting her period is a normal part of life and there is nothing about it to fear. If she never inquires about it and you start noticing body changes, casually bring it up.

If you sense that she is uncomfortable discussing it with you, try beginning the conversation in the car when the two of you are alone. This is a great time, since you don't have to sit and talk face to face.

Q: Every time I bring up menstruation my daughter tells me she doesn't want to talk about it. What should I do?

A: Definitely don't force the issue, and also make sure you are not projecting your nervousness about the subject onto your daughter. Kids are very aware of subjects that make you uncomfortable. At a minimum, admit your own discomfort with the subject if it exists. Reassure her that it is normal for people to not want to talk about periods, but that it is important to know about it.

Buy her a book like *My Body, Myself* that simply explains the process to her or **go over Menstruation 101** in this book (pp 17 - 24). A month or so after you have given her the information, ask her if she has any questions or if she would like to talk about it. If she doesn't, reassure her that she can always come to you with questions or concerns about her cycle. Again, try not to force her, but equip her with the information that she needs.

If your daughter is embarrassed about talking candidly about the subject, especially around her father or any other males in the household, come up with code names for her to use to inform you about the issue. A common one we used is "it's that time of the month" or "my friend Flo is in town......" Come up with something that's uniquely yours, something that the two of you share only with one another. You'll also find this strengthens your communication and mother/daughter bond.

Q: How can I teach my daughter to successfully deal with the onset of her menstruation?

A: A great suggestion is to help her to keep a menstrual diary.

Q: Sounds interesting. What should a menstrual diary contain?

A: A menstrual diary is a record of when your periods come, how long they are, how heavy they are and what symptoms are associated with your cycle. There are many ways to do this. Even a basic calendar or school planner can be used. I often give girls a simple chart to keep track like the one on page 38. There are some on-line menstrual diaries as well.

I personally think it is a good idea, especially when you first start having periods, to keep track of your cycles to make sure that they are normal. A menstrual diary often helps identify trends such as menstrual related headache and symptoms of premenstrual syndrome. If you need to see a health care provider for problems with your period, the diary can be extremely useful in identifying problems. Remember it does not need to be anything fancy and it can be in your own special code as long as you can interpret it.

TABLE TALK

A Beginning Conversation on Menstruation: Bringing up your own period can be a great way to start the conversation.

MY MONTHLY MENSTRUAL CALENDAR

YEAR: _____

MONTH	1	2	3	4	5	6	7	8	9	10	11	12	13	14	15	16	17	18	19	20	21	22	23	24	25	26	27	28	29	30	31
JANUARY																															
FEBRUARY																															
MARCH																															
APRIL																															
MAY																															
JUNE																															
JULY																															
AUGUST																															
SEPTEMBER																															
OCTOBER																															
NOVEMBER																															
DECEMBER																															

Use this calendar to mark down when you get your period each month. After a few months you should notice a pattern. This will help you know what days to expect your period to start.

(Connie (Mom), sitting in the family room; Brandy (daughter) comes in and sits down with Mom.)

Connie: I am feeling like I am about to start my cycle...

Brandy: Thanks for that one, Mom. Like I needed to know that.

Connie: Does that subject make you uncomfortable?

Brandy: Sort of.

Connie: Why?

Brandy: It just does.

Connie: I remember feeling uncomfortable about the subject when I was young, especially as my body was beginning to change. And then, when you add hormones to the mix, it can be overwhelming. Your body is looking more mature.

Brandy: Yea, my friend Carrie already started her cycle.

CONVERSATION STARTERS

Conversation starters on the subject of menstruation.

For daughters:

• Bring up the fact that a friend has started her period.

• Mention the fact that you may need a bra.

• When watching television, if an advertisement for feminine products pops up, ask questions. Or just make a comment.

• If your mom mentions anything about her period, use it as a starter.

• Just be straight forward and tell your mom you have some questions about menstruation.

For moms:

• If your daughter's body is maturing, make notice of the fact.

• If she needs to start wearing a bra, discuss shopping for one.

• If you are on your period, bring it up by mentioning that you are on your period. Let her know you consider it a natural part of being a woman, and is something you consider worthy of conversation.

• When her school shows "the film" or her health class is discussing menstruation, ask her if there are any questions.

• When you purchase feminine hygiene products, do it when your daughter is with you.

• No matter how young she may be, if she has any questions answer honestly.

Or how about this: If neither of you can think of a way to jump start a conversation, number the Q & A items in this chapter. Randomly select one by picking numbers out of a hat, by rolling some dice, or by closing your eyes and dropping a finger somewhere on the page. Read the Q&A out loud; then move on to something else. Make it into a "silly" game so the conversation doesn't get too heavy.

CHAPTER 2
_____

"But I'm not sick. Do I really need to see a doctor?"

ROUTINE HEALTH CARE

Routine health care is an ever present factor in a woman's life. It is important to develop conversations on an ongoing basis about routine health care. We stress the fact that it's always more difficult to start this discussion *after* a crisis has emerged, rather than before.

There is a lot of emotional preparation that is needed for a girl before going into her first gynecological exam. Eliminating the mystery of what is done during an exam will help lower the tension and fear of the first visit.

Here's a way to break it down.

Let's begin with what a *well woman exam* is exactly. A typical well woman exam includes a *personal health history, family health history,* and a *physical examination.* In our office we have you fill out an extensive questionnaire prior to being put in a room. It is *very important* that you answer the questions as honestly as possible, for by doing so you can be assured of the best care. Don't worry: whatever you answer will be kept strictly confidential.

The *personal history* includes questions about your past medical history: any illnesses, surgeries, medications (including non-prescription, over-the-counter, and herbal remedies). A menstrual history includes when you started your cycle, how often they come, how heavy your cycles are, and any problems you may experience such as cramps or irregular cycles. Your menstrual chart developed in the previous chapter (page 38) may come in handy here.

A *sexual history* includes questions about whether you have had sex, number of partners, sexual orientation, pain with intercourse, and any concerns or problems regarding sexual activity. A *social history* includes questions about alcohol, drug use, or smoking.

The *pelvic exam* comes next, and includes a *speculum exam* and a *bimanual exam.* A speculum is a small metal or plastic instrument that is inserted into the vagina. When a speculum is gently widened, it allows me to visualize the cervix, the tip of the uterus. In order to facilitate this part of the exam your feet are placed in the stirrups, and you have to move your buttocks to the end of the table so that they hang off the edge a bit. Having your bottom hang off the end of the table slightly and letting your legs fall open helps relax your vagina and makes the exam more comfortable. This exam won't be comfortable but should **not** be painful.

When the speculum is in the vagina, a Pap smear will be done. A Pap smear is a test to look for early signs of cervical cancer. If sexually transmitted disease testing is required, it will be done at this time as well. The speculum is then removed, and the bimanual exam is done to assess the size, tenderness, and mobility of the uterus and to evaluate ovaries for their size and tenderness.

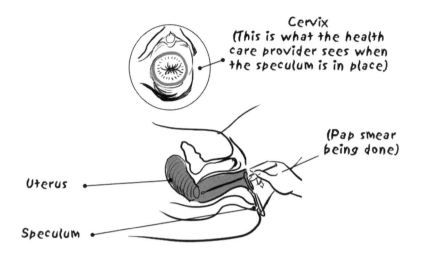

Cervix
(This is what the health
care provider sees when
the speculum is in place)

(Pap smear
being done)

Uterus

Speculum

First Part
The Speculum Exam

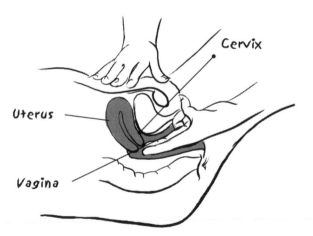

Cervix

Uterus

Vagina

Second Part
The Bimanual Exam

The bimanual part of the exam is done by having the provider insert two fingers into the vagina and gently pressing over the uterus and ovaries. If a young girl is so tense that she just cannot relax and she is not sexually active, I will bring her back in a few months and try the exam again. A health care provider will take every measure to not traumatize a young girl for a Pap smear, especially a virgin. A girl who has had consensual intercourse should be able to relax enough for an exam. *Remember this should not be painful, but you will never look forward to a pelvic exam.*

Last but not least is the *physical exam.* It starts with a look at your skin and the membranes of your eyes and mouth, followed by a check-up from top to bottom. This includes feeling for lymph nodes in the neck and for your thyroid gland — a small gland at the base of the neck that normally moves up and down when you swallow, so you will be asked to swallow while we press on your throat. Next we will move on to listening to your heart and lungs with a stethoscope. Then on to the breast exam: you will be taught how to do a self breast exam in both sitting and standing positions. Then, with you lying down on your back, we'll feel your liver and abdomen. We try our very best to keep you as covered as possible to preserve modesty. As women's health care specialists, we work hard to be respectful, matter-of-fact, and accepting throughout the entire exam process.

Most women have mixed feelings about their yearly well woman exam. The procedure is uncomfortable, but a part of growing up is doing what must be done, even if we don't want to or it makes us uncomfortable. It is best to go into your first exam emotionally and mentally prepared. After the first time, the next one will be a piece of cake.

A 16-year-old girl comes into the office with her mother. Together they fill out the health questionnaire; the girl denies any sexual activity, menstrual problems, or any other health concerns. The mother is doing all of the talking for the young girl, answering questions even before they are asked. The more her mom insists on her having an exam, the quieter and angrier the girl seems. She sits on the table looking very upset to be in the office in the first place.

Finally, I ask the mom to step out of the room while I talk with her daughter. She reluctantly leaves the room. The daughter tells me that her mom is insisting on her having an exam even though she does not feel like she needs it. She definitely does not WANT it. I reassure her that no exam would take place on that day and, therefore, she needs to try to relax so that I can make sure that nothing else needs to be done at that visit.

I carefully question her about possible sexual abuse but don't get any indication of that happening. She opens up slightly, but I remain committed to NOT doing the exam. Nothing she tells me makes me change my mind about doing an exam. Even if she tells me she is having sex and needs a Pap test, I won't do it today for she is not emotionally prepared to have it done.

I offer the girl my card and tell her that she can call me with any problems or questions. It is clear that the relationship between mother and daughter is strained and has little chance of improving by sheer force. I bring the mother back into the room and commend her on establishing a relationship with a women's health provider. A connection with a provider is critical to routine health care. I also tell her that no exam needs to be done today. We do discuss heath care guidelines, such as taking a calcium supplement. The mom appears slightly upset, but I reiterate the reasons to do an exam and the down side of forcing an exam when her daughter is not emotionally prepared. We talk together about what the future exam would entail, and when would be an appropriate time to pursue it.

The mother and daughter leave, but do come back later for a routine well woman exam. At this appointment, the daughter comes in appearing much less angry. She feels like she already has a bit of a connection, knows what to expect, and is more talkative. We proceed with the complete well-woman exam.

DAUGHTER QUESTIONS

Routine Health Visits. Daughters, let's get some of your questions out of the way so you can better understand the ins and outs of routine health care for women.

Q: At what age do I need to visit a gynecologist for a routine exam?

A: When I mention *routine,* that means you are experiencing no problems and have no targeted concerns. There are many different guidelines regarding this question; however, I go by the guidelines set up by American College of Obstetrics and Gynecology (ACOG). Prior to May 2006, they had stated that you go for your first *routine* gynecological exam at age 21 or within three years of becoming sexually active. They revised that to say that girls should have their first visit to a gynecologist between the ages of 13 and 15.

The visit is for the adolescent to begin to establish a relationship with a women's health care provider. That relationship with a health care provider is important so that when a problem pops up or when it is time for a well woman exam, you will already have met the person who will examine you. A pelvic exam probably won't be done, but it is an excellent time for girls to be educated about their bodies and about preventative heath care. It's also a good time for the health care provider to answer any questions or address any concerns a young girl might have.

Q: But I'm too embarrassed to talk about these things...

A: Remember that health care providers are rarely surprised by anything you might tell them. The best patient-provider relationships are ones based on honesty and full disclosure, and sensitive discussions are non-judgmental. The main goal of most good health care professionals is to help you, and the best way to accomplish that is with a complete and truthful health history.

A family history is important in evaluating potential risks that may be passed on through inheritance. For example, your mom having had breast cancer at a young age may change how early we might screen you for the same condition. Ask your parents and siblings before you go for a check up if there is any important family history that should be passed along at the visit.

Q: How often do I need to have a routine gynecological exam?

A: Once you have had your first exam, like we talked about earlier, you should have a routine exam every year. If you have an abnormal Pap test your provider may want to see you more often.

Q: Will I have to have blood tests when I go for a check up?

A: A well-woman exam for a healthy girl who is sexually active with no complaints should only include blood testing that screens for a sexually transmitted disease (STD), such as an AIDS test, syphilis, and hepatitis testing. Otherwise, there are no routine blood tests that are done. Many providers order urine tests to screen for a bladder infection. Some screen for anemia with a complete blood count, but that is rare.

Remember, if you have any more questions, talk to your mother. She can help you understand the process and what will happen. The importance of these doctor visits is to make them *routine*. It is important for every woman young and old to have these exams done once a year. These exams help to point out any problems that may be going on with your body.

Q: Are you sure they have to touch me? I just don't want anyone poking at my body

A: We do everything possible to make you feel comfortable. You have no need to feel embarrassed and you should not feel pain. Yes, we will need to check your body to make sure you do not have any medical problems that need to be addressed, but we will not pull any surprises on you. Part of the reason we are writing this book is so that you and your mother can talk together about what to expect in a routine well-woman exam, and you can prepare yourselves for it. The two of you can decide together when is the best time for you to visit a health care provider.

Common gynecological problems in teens. Girls, lets move on to a discussion of gynecological issues we see quite frequently in our office. Moms, listen in, since many of these questions may be exceptional conversation starters. First there may be ***ovarian problems*** the doctor may need to assess.

Q: My friend was diagnosed with ovarian cysts. What are ovarian cysts? They sound pretty bad.

A: Well, as we described in the menstruation section, your ovaries are small little organs located on each side of your uterus. Ovarian cysts are small fluid filled sacs that develop in or on the ovary. They are not as bad as they sound and are actually quite common. There are several types of ovarian cysts. By far the most common ones that we see in young girls are *functional cysts*. Most of the time, they are harmless and go away without any intervention. However, they can cause a great deal of discomfort. Other types are less common and are rarely cancerous, but further work-up could be necessary.

Q: Why are they so common?

A: Since functional cysts come from the common process of ovulation, they are most usually what we will find. There are two types of functional cysts: *follicular cysts* and *luteal cysts*.

Here comes that *Menstruation 101* again. Remember that in the first half of the cycle, follicles form prior to ovulation. One of the follicles can continue to grow and form a small cyst. Many girls form these and never know they have them, but if a cyst becomes too large it can cause pain. If a cyst ruptures and the fluid comes out into the pelvis, it can be even more painful. Fluid that leaks into the pelvis causes an inflammation that can hurt for a few days.

The second type of functional cyst is the luteal cyst that comes after ovulation. A luteal cyst comes from a corpus luteum that continues to grow. It does not continue to produce hormones, but it can get big and painful or rupture like the follicular cyst. Luteal cysts may be uncomfortable — even painful, but are not dangerous and usually disappear on their own.

Q: How do you cure ovarian cysts?

A: Most ovarian cysts will go away without any intervention at all. Since most are related to the function of the ovaries, in a cycle or two they generally are gone. Many times, I will put a girl on the birth control pill for at least three months, which will allow the ovaries to take a break and heal. The pill gives the body the hormones that the ovaries would make, so the ovaries do not have to work (kind of like resting a sprained ankle!).

After a few months, if a girl does not want to take the pill any longer, I will take her off and see if the cysts reoccur. Rarely, an ovarian cyst needs to be surgically removed, but only if it is very large or it is felt that the ovary is twisted. The other, even less common, reason to remove a cyst is if there is a concern for bleeding occurring in the abdomen. This is very rare, but is important to identify. With abdominal bleeding, you would usually feel light-headed and nauseated, and have severe belly pain.

Q: How will a health care provider know that I have an ovarian cyst?

A: Most of the time, the best way to diagnose an ovarian cyst is with an abdominal ultrasound. A vaginal exam is usually not necessary unless the abdominal ultrasound can not see the ovaries. This generally only occurs if someone is obese. What the radiologist looks for during the ultrasound are fluid-filled little cysts on the ovary or free fluid in the pelvis. The radiologist will measure how big the cyst is or how much fluid is in the pelvis.

Vaginal Problems. Now, there are also *vaginal problems* that may need to be addressed by an OB/GYN.

Q: I always have a vaginal discharge. Is this abnormal?

A: Vaginal discharge is normal. Ask any menopausal woman who has vaginal dryness, and she will tell you that *having no* discharge is much more uncomfortable than *having* a vaginal discharge. Hormone production causes a discharge that will change throughout the month. For instance, around ovulation, discharge gets heavier and more noticeable. Clear to white discharge in varying amounts is okay. Discharge is not normal if it itches, burns, or has a fishy type of odor. In these situations, you need to see a health care provider to look for an infection.

Q: How are vaginal infections diagnosed?

A: Vaginal infections are diagnosed by finding out about the history of the abnormal discharge: how long you have had it, what the discharge looks like, whether it itches or burns, and whether it has an odor. Then we need to get a sample of the discharge. If you are very nervous and you are not sexually active I will not use a speculum. I'll just insert a small Q-tip® into the vagina to get a sample. If you are sexually active or if you can relax, I will do a speculum exam — it makes it easier for me to get sufficient sample material.

After I obtain the sample, I do something called a *wet prep* where I make a smear on the slide and use a microscope to actually look at the type of cells that are there. If you have yeast, I can see yeast buds and yeast hyphae. If you have BV (Bacterial Vaginosis), I will see what are called *clue cells*. I also do a test called a *whiff test* where I put a chemical on the slide that produces the fishy type smell. There are also some tests that are run in a machine, looking for the harmful bacteria. These tests sometimes are more accurate.

Q: So if I have a discharge that has a fishy odor, I should be concerned?

A: When you have a fishy-type odor, you probably have a vaginal infection called Bacterial Vaginosis or BV. This is common, and you can get it without being sexually active. First of all, your vagina, like your mouth, has bacteria. Bacteria help in keeping your vagina healthy by getting rid of more harmful bacteria that shouldn't be there. When you have BV, it is an overgrowth of the wrong kind of bacteria. This imbalance in the vagina can be due to a variety of causes. Antibiotics are famous for causing BV as well other vaginal infections. The antibiotics kill off the protective bacteria and the wrong type can then overgrow. You can get BV other ways too, including through sexual activity, having too much moisture from sitting around in wet clothes, or taking too many baths.

A 15-year-old girl, Alyssa, who was not sexually active, came to the office because she was having constant vaginal discharge. Her sexual history was negative; she had never had sex. Her menstrual history was normal. She continued telling me she thought she had picked up some sort of disease, perhaps from a public rest room. I asked her to tell me her symptoms. She said that she always had this sticky discharge and was afraid to tell anyone, but finally told her mom. I asked her if it smelled or had an odor and she denied both.

I told her that I could check it by inserting a cotton swab into the vagina to test the discharge by looking at it under the microscope. I showed her the normal results under the microscope. She still argued that the discharge was not normal — she just knew something was wrong with her. I explained that the reason she had vaginal discharge was because her body was producing hormones that cause vaginal secretions. The amount varies from girl to girl and throughout the month. I spent the rest of the visit reassuring her that discharge was normal, and helping her to know how to identify discharge that might not be normal. She asked the same question again, just to make sure I hadn't changed my mind, misspoken, or tricked her. The visit was intense. However, she seemed immensely relieved when she left. For years she had secretly worried she had some sort of disease.

Q: What about douching to clean yourself out?

A: Bad idea. Douching can cause you to wash away the protective bacteria, so there is almost never a good reason to douche. The word "douche" means to wash or soak in French. Douching is washing or cleaning out the vagina (also called the birth canal) with water or other mixtures of fluids. Usually douches are prepackaged mixes of water and vinegar, baking soda, or iodine. Women can buy these products at drug and grocery stores. The mixtures usually come in a bottle and can be squirted into the vagina through a tube or nozzle.

Women douche because they mistakenly believe it gives many benefits. *In reality, douching may do more harm than good.* By washing away the protective bacteria, you can then increase the chances of growing the wrong kind of bacteria (BV). Often you cannot exactly pinpoint how you got it, but BV is generally easy to diagnose and cure. The best and most common treatment is an antibiotic called metronidazole or Flagyl®. Generally, you take it twice a day for 7-10 days. There is a one time oral regimen but the longer regimens work better. This medicine will make you extremely ill if you drink any alcohol at all while you are being treated. There are also several vaginal preparations that range from a one-dose therapy to a five-day therapy.

Q: I have a white, clumpy discharge that itches a lot and looks like cottage cheese. Should I go to the doctor?

A: This is probably another very common vaginal infection called a *yeast infection*. Everyone has seen the commercials on the radio, TV, or in a magazine for yeast infection treatments. This condition can be extremely uncomfortable and you can even get pubic swelling along with the itching and discharge. Yeast infections are most commonly caused by antibiotics killing off the good bacteria and allowing the yeast to overgrow, similar to what occurs with BV.

There are several treatments, both prescription and non-prescription. If you have never had one before and are not certain what you have, I would see your health care provider first. Over-the-counter products like vaginal creams work frequently, especially for the most common form of yeast called Candida.

If you are sure that you have a yeast infection, there are non-prescription preparations available at the pharmacy. They tend to be vaginal suppositories or creams that you use for one to seven days. I prefer a 7-day cream or suppository, for the ones you use for fewer days can be very irritating. The other problem with these creams is that they only treat one strain of yeast.

The prescription medication available from your health care provider is either an oral medication or topical creams and suppositories that are stronger than over-the-counter or non-prescription preparations. Most girls like the oral medication that can be given in a single dose, but I think the 2-dose kind works better. The creams and vaginal suppositories are useful for one to seven days. The single-dose prescription works very well. The creams treat all three types of yeast.

Q: Are vaginal infections ever sexually transmitted?

A: That all depends. Yeast infections generally are not sexually transmitted, and we rarely ever treat a sexual partner for yeast. Bacterial Vaginosis is considered by some to be an STD, although I have treated virgins for BV — especially ones who douche. We generally do not treat partners for BV and research rarely suggests benefit by doing so. That is another reason I have a hard time calling it an STD. There is another vaginal infection called trichomonas or "trich" that is generally sexually transmitted. We'll talk about it later when we cover STDs.

Q: I keep having recurrent vaginal infections. Is there anything I can do to prevent them?

A: There are some girls who do start having chronic vaginal infections and it can get tricky. The main thing to do if this occurs is to start looking for patterns. If every time you go swimming you end up sitting around in a wet bathing suit, try to change that behavior. Some infections go along with hormonal changes, so you should keep track of your cycles and look to see if there is a pattern as to when they occur each month.

When chronic vaginal infections keep reoccurring, we sometimes start a birth control pill, or change the pill if you are already on one. If you douche, stop. The other culprit can be deodorant tampons or pads, perfumed soaps, and chemicals in laundry detergent that cause irritation and inflammation that is often confused with a yeast infection.

Other health problems. Let's talk about some other common health problems we encounter. Many of these may be things you've heard your friends talk about.

Q: I was visiting my cousin. When we were changing, she told me that I needed to shave because I was too hairy in the pubic area. Now, after shaving, I got the worst bumps. Why?

A: First of all, you don't have to shave because someone thinks you're too hairy. I know a lot of young girls do shave to accommodate clothing. I don't have a problem with people shaving the pubic area, but I also see a lot of skin irritation related to shaving in the pubic area. I think waxing is less irritating.

It is important to use a new razor or blade every time you shave. Sharp blades reduce the irritation. Also, there are some after-shaving creams and gels to decrease irritation. Finally, some people do use depilatory products, but they can also irritating.

Q: Depilatory? Sounds scary....

A: No... depilatory is just a fancy name for hair removal. These can be bought at your store where beauty products are sold. There are many types of creams, lotions, or waxes that all remove hair. Some of them are easier to use than others and some can be irritating. You'll have to experiment if you want to go the hair-removal route.

Q: My friend has endometriosis. What is that, and how do I know if I have it?

A: It is estimated that 25% of adolescents who present to providers with chronic pelvic pain will have endometriosis. The most important part of the physiology of endometriosis is that menstrual tissue from the uterine lining comes up out of the fallopian tubes (retrograde menstruation) instead of down through the vagina, and this tissue implants in the different parts of the pelvis and abdomen. After the uterine tissue implants, a complex immunologic reaction occurs, causing the pain with menstrual period or even pelvic pain when not on a period.

It is very hard to diagnose endometriosis with complete certainty without doing surgery. Even with surgery, though, the microscopic endometriosis that causes significant pain may not be found. Therefore, to diagnose endometriosis we end up just making sure that there is no other cause for the pain. For example, the best way to be sure there isn't an ovarian cyst or other problem is through exam and pelvic ultrasound.

Often when a young girl comes in with pelvic pain and both the exam and the ultrasound are normal, the first line of treatment is birth control pills. Many girls who take the pill will get significant relief or at least stop the progression of pain. If that doesn't control the pain, then there are other medications that can be tried. Often exploratory surgery will be done to see if there are visible signs of endometriosis.

Q: I have noticed some nipple discharge. Should I be concerned?

A: You definitely need to see your health care provider to make sure it is normal. Nipple discharge happens for a number of reasons, with the most common being pregnancy or breast feeding. But, if you are neither pregnant nor nursing, the most common type of nipple discharge is a milky discharge often caused by a growth on the pituitary gland. The pituitary is responsible for the production of a hormone called prolactin which helps make your body produce milk. A small, almost always benign growth on the pituitary can cause an elevation of the prolactin level causing you to begin to produce milk. Other common causes can be an underactive thyroid gland or certain medications.

Another type of commonly reported nipple discharge is a clear liquid that sometimes can be squeezed out of the nipple. Sometimes, with a lot of nipple stimulation you can get clear fluid, but again you need a breast exam.

Finally, some people will present to the office with bloody or greenish nipple discharge. This is rare but can indicate a cyst or an infection. Most of the time, these conditions are not cancer; however, you will want to see a health care provider to determine the cause and if any treatment is necessary.

A 17-year-old-girl named Mary came into the office because she noticed she had wet spots on her bra when she took it off. When she squeezed her nipple she noticed white fluid coming out that resembled milk. She told me her periods had become irregular over the past six months, often skipping two to three periods. She stated she had never been sexually active and could not possibly be pregnant.

When she came into the office I examined her breast for lumps. There were none. When I pressed on her nipples, white liquid came out. I put some of the fluid on a slide to send to the lab to look at the cells. I also sent some blood tests out to check prolactin level, which is a hormone that can cause breasts to make milk. When I got her blood test back her prolactin level was elevated to 75 (A normal level in a nonbreastfeeding woman is 25 or less).

I sent her to an endocrinologist who diagnosed a pituitary adenoma, a small benign growth on her pituitary that was causing her to produce milk. They used various medications to shrink the growth, and the last time I spoke to her the milky breast discharge had stopped and she was doing well. She will continue to be followed by the endocrinologist as well.

Q: I have found a breast lump. How likely is it to be cancer?

A: It is very unlikely to be breast cancer. In fact, I can say that with greater than 99% certainty for women under 30. It is important to learn how to check your breast so that if you have a new or different lump you will know. Many girls find breast exams difficult since breast tissue can normally be very lumpy and women don't know how a suspicious lump feels. When you have a breast lump, it usually will feel different than the other parts of your breast. I describe it as when you come across a pebble in sand, you don't have to look at the sand but you know that there is something different.

Any time you find or see something different in your breast, you should see your provider for a breast exam. Most breast lumps in young girls are called *fibroadenomas*. These are benign lumps that occur commonly in young women. They are mobile, round lumps of varying sizes. The other type of breast lump that occurs less frequently but can occur in this age group is a cyst due to fibrocystic breast disease.

Mammograms on young girls to look for breast cancer are often useless, so I usually send girls with lumps straight to a breast specialist for an ultrasound test and exam. Often, these benign breast lumps are just followed by the breast specialist, unless they are growing or become painful. Generally I do not suggest screening mammograms until the age of 40 unless there is a strong family history for breast cancer that occurred in the mother or sisters. In that case, I often recommend that you see a breast specialist on an annual basis once you are over 30. We cannot keep you from developing breast cancer, but early detection is certainly the goal.

Q: How and when do I do breast self exam?

A: The best time to do breast self exam is the week after your period begins. Remember you start your period because hormone levels drop and at other times in your cycle hormone stimulation can make your breast feel lumpy. The age to begin self breast exam is age 20. However, I believe it is never too early to know your body. Here are the self breast exam guidelines we recommend, which follow those outlined by the American Cancer Society.

How to Examine Your Breasts

Lie down and place your left arm behind your head. It's best to do the exam while lying down, not standing up. When you lie down the breast tissue spreads evenly over the chest wall, making it much easier to feel all the breast tissue.

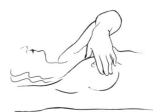

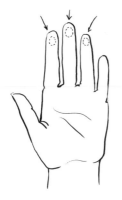

Use the pads of fingers on your right hand to feel for lumps in the left breast. Check the entire breast and armpit area. Use overlapping circular motions of the finger pads to feel the breast tissue.

Try three different levels of pressure to feel all the breast tissue. Light pressure is needed to feel the tissue closest to the skin; medium pressure to

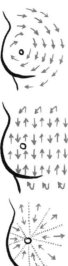

feel a little deeper; and firm pressure to feel the tissue closest to the chest and ribs. If you're not sure how hard to press, talk with your mother, doctor or nurse.

Move around the breast in an up and down pattern. It's easiest to start by imagining a line drawn straight down your side from the underarm, then move across the breast to the middle of the chest bone (sternum or breastbone). Be sure to check the entire breast area going down until you feel only ribs and up to the neck or collar bone (clavicle).

There are three patterns you can use to examine your breast: the circular, the up-and-down, and the wedge patterns. Use the pattern that is easiest for you, and use the same pattern every month.

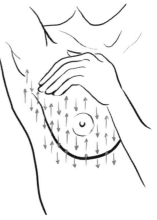

Some researchers suggest that the up and down (vertical) pattern is the most effective pattern for covering the entire breast without missing any breast tissue.

Repeat the exam on your right breast, using the finger pads of the left hand.

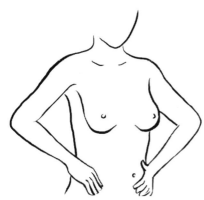

While standing in front of a mirror with your hands pressing firmly down on your hips, look at your breasts for any changes of size, shape, contour, dimpling, or redness or scaliness of the nipple or breast skin. (The pressing down on the hips position contracts the chest wall muscles and enhances any breast changes.) It is normal if your right and left breasts do not match exactly.

Examine each underarm while sitting up or standing and with your arm only slightly raised so you can

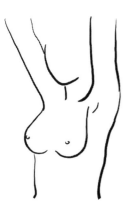

easily feel in this area. Raising your arm straight up tightens the tissue in this area and makes it difficult to examine.

Remember to do the same thing each month at the same time in your cycle. Check both breasts.

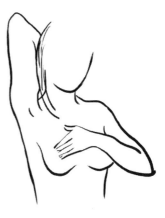

MOM QUESTIONS

Girls, you're not the only ones with questions about *routine health care* and *gynecologists*. Listen in on some of your mother's questions. You may be surprised to find out that they are similar to yours.

Q: My daughter needs to visit a gynecologist. What can I do to prepare her for the exam?

A: The most important way to prepare your daughter for her exam is to reassure her that it probably won't be as bad as she thinks it will be. Discuss what is involved with the exam, but remind her that the more she can relax, the easier the exam will be. Acknowledge to her that it is uncomfortable, and that sitting on a table naked, only covered by a large paper gown, can certainly make her feel quite vulnerable. Let her know that she can discuss any problem with her provider, no matter how awkward it may seem. That is what providers do all the time. Also, put her in charge of the decision on whether she wants you to stay in the room during the exam or not. Abide by her wishes.

Q: How do I find the best health care provider for a first time gynecological exam for my teenage daughter?

A: To find a provider who is especially good with a girl's first exam, I recommend starting by talking to your friends, family physician, and even your own gynecologist. Your friends with daughters around the age as yours may already have a good person they would be happy to suggest. Since a friend may be someone who knows you and your daughter well, this can be a great resource.

Your family physician probably is well versed in the local medical community and can recommend people based on personal knowledge of both you and the providers to whom he or she refers patients. In my practice, many women have their own gynecologist, which is a great place to start for your own daughter. Others opt to see someone based on a referral from their women's health care provider.

Q: My 14-year-old daughter was having problems with her period so I took her to my gynecologist. To my surprise, my gynecologist asked me to leave the room while she talked to her. Should I be upset that she asked me to leave the room?

A: Not at all. I almost always try to get a few minutes with an adolescent without her parent present so that I can make sure that there is nothing a young girl is not telling me simply because she doesn't want her mom to hear. I generally talk to both mother and daughter together. I will use that joint time to tell them both that to provide the best care to the patient I need an opportunity to talk to her alone. I explain that it gives the young woman a chance to ask a question that she might be afraid to ask in front of her parent and to allow her to take control of her own health care. I also reassure both of them that it is important to allow a young woman to have a sense of privacy because that says to her that you trust her. I also tell them both that if I feel that the patient is in danger I will definitely tell the parent; otherwise, I will try to establish a relationship that is between the patient and health care provider. Most people are very happy to go along with this approach.

Q: My daughter is 16 and sexually active, and has been to the gynecologist. Does she still need to see her pediatrician?

A: Yes, she does. Most gynecologists do little general care such as strep tests for sore throats or treatment for the flu. It is also important to see your pediatrician for routine vaccinations, especially before going to college. If your daughter does not want to continue to see her pediatrician, it is reasonable to have a family doctor for routine non-gynecological problems.

Q: My daughter was placed on birth control pills to shrink an ovarian cyst. Will she have to stay on the pill indefinitely?

A: First of all, the pill doesn't "shrink" the cyst, but it does allow the ovaries to take a break and heal. And no, she will not need to stay on the pills permanently unless she is chronically forming painful cysts. Generally, I will encourage a young girl to stay on them for three months and then see what happens to her symptomatic cysts.

Q: My daughter had an ovarian cyst. How likely is she to have more cysts?

A: No one can accurately predict this, but if she chronically gets pelvic pain that is thought to be due to ovarian cysts, staying or getting on birth control pills can be very helpful.

Q: My daughter keeps having recurrent vaginal infections. Should I be concerned that she is sexually active?

A: No, you should not be concerned that it automatically means she is sexually active. The most important thing to do when your daughter gets frequent vaginal infections is to be certain that the diagnosis is correct and you have completely treated the problem. Many infections are inadequately treated based on symptoms alone and may need confirmatory testing. We get a lot of patients who come in telling us they have chronic yeast infections, and when we do the wet prep, they don't have yeast at all! In these cases, the girls can have inflammation from chronic itching, and the key intervention is to break the itch cycle. In other cases, the infection is never completely cleared and a different treatment is needed.

There are reasons why girls get these types of infection and they generally are not related to sexual activity.

Nancy was on an antibiotic medication for her skin. Indeed, it helped the skin condition. She later came into the women's health clinic complaining of chronic yeast infection. It took quite some time, with repeated trips to the clinic, to figure out why she chronically kept getting infections. Revisiting the medical history, it became apparent that the antibiotic medication prescribed for her acne was the culprit. Both Nancy and her mother had innocently assumed that on the questionnaire, when asked about "current and past medications," the questions referred to gynecological medications. Skin medications would, of course, be irrelevant, or so they thought! Even though the information seems trivial, a complete and thorough answer to medical history and personal health history questions is invaluable to promptly resolving recalcitrant infections.

Q: Should I encourage my daughter to cleanse herself differently to prevent infections?

A: A mild soap like Dove® is fine, but only wash externally. Skip soaps that have deodorants and perfumes since they can cause external irritation and itching. The vagina is a self cleansing organ and washing too vigorously can get rid of the natural protection that is meant to be there. Most vaginal infections are not due to being unclean.

Q: Breast cancer runs in my family. Does my daughter need to be screened earlier than average?

A: I'll tell you the same thing I told your daughter a few pages back. Generally I do not suggest screening mammograms until the age of 40 unless you have a strong family history for breast cancer. Strong family history for breast cancer means breast cancer that has affected your mother or sisters. In this case, I often recommend that you see a breast specialist once a year after you are over 30. We can not keep you from developing breast cancer, but early detection is certainly the goal.

Q: My daughter has been complaining of left breast pain for the last three weeks. Should I take her to see her health care provider?

A: First of all, this is a great time to teach your daughter breast self exam and visual inspection. You might look together at the section in this book on doing an exam (pages 57 - 59), or even visit a web site together like that of the American Cancer Society.

I never think it is a bad idea if you are having problems with your breast to see a health care provider to make sure that there is not a significant problem. However, breast pain is usually not a sign of cancer. The first question I would ask her is "When is your period going to start?" If her pain is present but she is about to have her cycle it is reasonable to wait until after her cycle and see if the pain decreases. Most breast pain or *mastodynia* in a young girl is related to hormonal stimulation to the breast tissue. Since the beginning of your period is signaled by a drop in hormones, often the pain will decrease after a cycle. Sometimes decreasing caffeine and adding 400 I.U. of Vitamin E can decrease breast pain.

If a girl seeks medical care for breast pain, a breast exam would be important. Assuming no lumps were found, it would be important to explain to the patient how hormone levels associated with her monthly cycle can affect breast pain, and to monitor the pain for a few cycles. Frequently that is sufficient reassurance for a young girl. A mammogram is rarely done in this age group since breast tissue is too dense in the developing breast. If a lump is found then the patient would be referred for an ultrasound.

TABLE TALK

Preparing for the First Gynecological Visit. (Tori, 15-year-old daughter, with severe cramps; Tori's mom, Kathy).

Kathy: I've noticed you're missing more activities because of cramps. They seem so much worse every month.

Tori: Yeah, each month they get even more painful.

Kathy: How do feel about going to see a gynecologist about your cramps getting more severe?

Tori: What? A gynecologist! Why?

Kathy: A gynecologist has more knowledge about what to do to help with your cramps.

Tori: But will she have to examine me? That scares me.

Kathy: She probably will not have to examine you. If she does, we won't do it at the first visit. This visit will allow you to meet your very own health care provider and decide if you need to visit more.

Conversation Starters

"Conversation Starters" on the subject of routine health care, and some recommended activities.

For moms:

1. I noticed that you are going through sanitary napkins very quickly. Are your periods really heavy?

2. You have missed a lot of activities related to cramps. Would you like to go to the doctor to see if there is anything we can do?

3. In your health class at school, do they teach breast self exam?

4. Would you like to go to a gynecologist, not for an exam, but to talk about things you need to know about your body and female health care? That way, if a problem develops, or if you have questions, you will already have a relationship with a health care provider.

5. You and your boyfriend have been spending a lot of time together. Do you have any questions that you might be more comfortable addressing to a health care provider? I would be happy to make an appointment for you.

For daughters:

1. If I had a female health problem would I go to my pediatrician or to your doctor?

2. Mom, every time my period comes I have bad breast pain ... I'm not sure I can tell if there is a problem.

3. Mom, did you have cramps when you were young, and what did you do for them?

4. When did you first go to a gynecologist?

5. When do I need to have my first female exam, and will it hurt?

CHAPTER 3

"How Do I Know If I've Got It?"

SEXUALLY TRANSMITTED DISEASES (STDs)

Everyday in our office we come in contact with someone who has a sexually transmitted disease (STD). Most often it is HPV *(human papillomavirus),* but in our teen population we also see quite a bit of herpes and Chlamydia. It is estimated that 13 million people in the United States are newly diagnosed each year with STDs. The good news is that during the last fifteen years there has been a decline in the number of STDs. This decline is attributed to the use of condoms. Still, even among very well educated people, we are always amazed at the number of cases of Chlamydia diagnosed every year. As these infections are preventable, we need to improve the education our youth are receiving about STDs.

The more adolescents we see who are diagnosed with sexually transmitted diseases, the more it becomes apparent how ill-equipped adolescents are when it comes to STDs. Many of the girls don't know what they are, much less what steps can be taken to prevent them, or to protect against them.

When we call a girl to tell her that she has an abnormal Pap smear, many times she's never heard of the human papillomavirus that can cause the abnormality and has no understanding what this means. Often times, she will tell me that she only has one partner; that, consequently, she could not possibly have HPV or any other STD.

Like most girls, she doesn't understand that she may have only one partner, but that one partner could have had one — or twenty — partners. He brings to her anything he has contracted through those partners. Often, when questioned about condom use she will tell me that she uses them, but when asked if she uses them *every* time the answer is most often "no." Condoms only offer protection if they are used *all* of the time. Even girls who have another girl as a partner can get an STD.

DAUGHTER QUESTIONS

STD Questions. Girls, let's turn to some questions we get all the time in our office. Don't be afraid to ask, because I can guarantee you that you're not the only one with your question. Moms, listen in, since you may find yourselves talking about these issues with your daughters.

Q: What is an STD? How do I know that I have one?

A: Every year, millions of people in the United States are diagnosed with sexually transmitted infections. A sexually transmitted disease is an infection that is spread through sexual contact. You don't need to have sexual intercourse to get a sexually transmitted infection. STDs are very contagious, and they are definitely "out there." Many STDs can be cured, but some cannot. Prevention is the best medicine.

Often, STDs don't have signs or symptoms and people have no idea they are infected. Nevertheless, the infection can be doing significant damage to your body, or be spread to someone else. As a child once said to me, "I am the boss of me," so please remember you are the boss of your body.

First off there's *human papillomavirus (HPV)*, a viral infection that is spread by intimate skin to skin contact. It lives in skin cells, especially in the vulva, vagina and cervix. There are more than 100 different strains of HPV. Some are not as dangerous to you, but some are. HPV is the leading cause of cervical cancer, vaginal cancer, vulvar cancer, genital warts, and some oral cancers. There is a small amount of evidence that it can cause cancer of the penis, but that is rare. The types of HPV that cause cancer are called "high risk" types.

It is estimated that eight out of ten people are infected with some type of HPV. More alarming, there are no early signs that you might have been infected with HPV. Genital warts are the most common symptom of HPV. Genital warts can be anywhere in the genital area, even down the thigh or near the anus.

Q: I think I have genital warts. How do I find out for sure, and how are they treated?

A: Genital warts are caused by the human papillomavirus infection and are also called *condyloma acuminata,* or *veneral warts.* Not all HPV infections will cause genital warts. The warts can be anywhere on the vulva, around the anus, inside the vagina, or even on the cervix. Most warts are soft, moist flesh colored lesions. Sometimes they have a *cauliflower* look; some are flat or raised. They can occur in a cluster or as just one or two warts.

The first step in treating warts is to see your health care provider to make sure they really are warts, which is usually done by looking at them. The treatment I most commonly recommend is a self-applied cream called *imiquimod cream.* The cream gets rid of warts very effectively and has the best track record for preventing reoccurrence. There are a few other self-applied treatments and even some solutions designed to be applied directly in the medical office. For the most part, they are moderately effective at getting rid of the warts.

If these treatments don't work I will occasionally surgically remove them using local anesthesia. The advantage to surgical removal is that the lab will examine the tissue removed for an accurate diagnosis. Other treatments that can be used are *cryosurgery* (freezing), *electrocautery* (burning), and *laser treatment.*

Q: Are genital warts just in girls, or can my boyfriend have them too?

A: On males, warts can be anywhere on the penis, scrotum, or anal area. Look: if you see anything, *stay away!* Understand that just because you are not having intercourse, it does not mean you cannot get infected, because HPV can be spread just by skin to skin contact. The risk factors associated with HPV are: first intercourse at an early age, large number of sexual partners for you or your partner, smoking, or having a problem with the immune system. Prevention is the best way to deal with HPV.

Q: I was told I have cervical dysplasia caused by HPV. How do you treat it, and can I get rid of it?

A: There are three levels of dysplasia: mild, moderate, and severe. The treatment will depend on the severity of the dysplasia. In years past it was believed that once you were infected with the HPV you would have the infection — forever. With the advent of the HPV DNA test that is done on a Pap smear, we now find people able to get to a point where the virus cannot be detected at all. For a girl with dysplasia, if she is in her twenties and practices low-risk sexual behavior, she has a 75 percent chance that her infection will clear in two to three years with no treatment at all.

Therefore, in *mild dysplasia,* there is often no treatment; just frequent follow-up Pap smears and DNA testing. If this is the treatment choice, it also is the time to reiterate the importance of limiting sexual partners and using condoms. Remember, having multiple sexual partners automatically places you in the high risk group. Some health care providers may opt to do cryosurgery, which involves chemically freezing the cervix with a small probe. This procedure lasts less than 10 minutes. The frozen tissue sloughs off, allowing new normal cells to grow back.

For *moderate dysplasia* cryotherapy is sometimes used, but frequently the treatment will be a *LEEP* (Loop Electrosurgical Excision Procedure). The procedure is generally done in the doctor's office with local anesthesia. This procedure allows the operator to take off millimeters of abnormal cervical tissue. The removed tissue is sent to the lab to determine whether all the abnormal cells were removed. Most women are back to typical activities in one to three days. After the procedure you may have cramping which usually ends by the next day. Vaginal discharge and spotting may occur for up to three weeks. It is important not to use tampons nor have sexual intercourse after the procedure, as directed by the person who did the LEEP.

For *severe dysplasia* a cone biopsy may be performed. It is generally done in the hospital under general anesthesia as an outpatient. A cone shaped biopsy is done on the cervix, allowing the more extensive abnormalities to be removed. Again, this tissue will be examined in the lab. Most women return to normal activity in about one week. There can be bleeding for up to one week, and vaginal discharge up to three weeks. Again, the same rules apply: nothing in the vagina until after your post-op check.

Q: Is there anything I can do to prevent HPV?

A: Just recently the FDA approved a vaccine that prevents the spread of four of the most common high risk types of HPV. These four types are responsible for 70% of the strains that cause cervical cancer and 90% of the types that cause genital warts.

The good news is that for young girls, if you stay healthy and practice low risk behavior, you can prevent or even clear infections. For girls who are between the ages of 9 and 26, get vaccinated! And always use condoms in new relationships.

HPV infection *is something I deal with just about everyday that I work. One case, however, stands out as one of the* *most difficult situations I have ever come across. A 15-year-old girl and her mother came into the office for an exam. The daughter claimed to have never been sexually active, either in the present or the past. I explained to the mother that since her daughter had not had sex, and since she was so young, she really did not need an exam. The mom insisted, however. She wanted to have the exam since they came from a family that had many genital malformations, and she wanted to be sure that "things were normal."*

When asked about the types of malformations, she was uncertain but insisted that she needed to know if everything was normal. I told her I could conduct an exam, but her daughter really didn't need a Pap. It was not called for. Again, the mom insisted. So I conceded. I agreed to do the Pap and exam. The young girl got through the exam just fine. In fact, she did not seem at all scared, bothered, or stressed by the exam which, frankly, I found very unusual.

Her Pap results showed moderate dysplasia and were positive for high risk human papillomavirus. I called the results to the mother to discuss the need for a colposcopy. She just kept telling me there must be a mistake, that her daughter was not sexually active, and the specimen must have gotten mixed up. I told her that was unlikely; however, we would take a look with the colposcope to verify that unlikely possibility. Daughter continued to deny sexual activity.

The colposcopy was consistent with the Pap test, and recommendations were for the patient to have a "leep." We never got to the root of the problem, however. They left without returning.

It haunts me to this day. Was there some sexual abuse that both the mother and patient were aware of but didn't speak of? Or was it that the daughter was sexually active and did not want her mother to know? Or did the mother know the daughter was sexually active and they just could not communicate about it, insisting instead that her daughter have an exam? Was it possible the medical results were misleading, not once, not twice, but three separate times? One thing is for sure: I am glad that I followed my gut and proceeded with the exam. At least with that information the mother and daughter had the opportunity to begin some "Table Talk."

Q: How does the HPV vaccine work, and should I get it?

A: For more than a decade, at every conference I attended there was discussion of a vaccine that was coming out "soon" to protect against the human papilloma virus. I would then go back to work to deal with overwhelming numbers of abnormal Pap smears in women of all ages and wish for this vaccine to hit the market as soon as possible.

When the vaccine came out in the United States and the controversy started, I was in shock. We had come out with a vaccine that protected women from *cervical cancer 70% of the time*, yet people began to make it into a moral issue, suggesting that it would encourage girls to have sex. The vaccine had been available in European countries for years. I often wondered if cancer of the penis happened as frequently as cervical abnormalities, would the same issues have arisen?

In discussing cancer prevention through vaccine use, abstinence always comes up as the substitute. Let's think about this for a minute. Most of the time, at least one person in the couple will not be a virgin, or at the very least will have had some type of intimate contact with another partner by the time marriage occurs. The statistics are staggering.

Second, even if you are a virgin at the time of marriage, the divorce rate in the US is 50%, so it is likely that one or both of you will have another partner in your lifetime. Third, what if you met the perfect man who had made a few poor choices when younger. Would you decide not to marry him in order to not risk cancer, or would you go ahead and marry him but risk cancer? Finally, the worst thought would be rape. Would you want to deal with cervical abnormalities as yet another part of this devastating ordeal? No one knows what is around the next bend in life. Even the most conservative person is likely to have more than one sexual partner in his or her lifetime.

Q: So you think the HPV vaccine is something I should get now?

A: YES, YES, YES! You should get the vaccine if your health care provider recommends that you receive the vaccine. Remember, this is a vaccine to prevent cancer, not the common cold. Even if you have come in contact with HPV it is still recommended that you receive the vaccine.

The HPV vaccine is purified inactive proteins from four of the most common high risk types of the virus. The body recognizes the inactive proteins of the virus and begins to make antibodies. These antibodies give you protection if you then come in contact with the virus.

The vaccine that is presently available is produced with the same technology as the hepatitis vaccine that every child receives at birth, and is very safe. The vaccine is recommended for girls between the ages of 9 and 26. It is best to receive the vaccine before becoming sexually active.

TABLE TALK

Table Talk Conversation on Doctor Visit for HPV vaccine. (Cindy, a 15-year-old girl riding in the car with her mother, Kathy; on their way to the pediatrician for a routine check up.)

Cindy: Will I have to have any shots today?

Kathy: I am not sure, but I'm going to ask your doctor about the HPV vaccine.

Cindy: HPV vaccine? My friends said that's only for people having sex. I'm not sexually active and I am going to abstain until I get married, so I don't really need to get the vaccine.

Kathy: I think that's great if you don't have sex until marriage, but I still want you to have the vaccine because it prevents cervical cancer 70% of the time.

Cindy: But if I don't have sex, I don't need it.

Kathy: First of all, how do you know that the person you marry won't have already been infected with the virus?

Cindy: I would only marry a virgin.

Kathy: You never know who you will fall in love with, and a lot of people have been infected with the HPV virus and don't even know it. Therefore, I think it is important to be vaccinated.

Cindy: Is it safe? Will it hurt?

Kathy: I can't promise that the shot won't hurt. It will probably hurt a bit. But cervical cancer or treatments after Pap test abnormalities would hurt a lot more.

Cindy: Can I wait till I am older when I am closer to having sex?

Kathy: I would rather you get the vaccination long before you become sexually active so that you will have the protection. That is the best way to avoid cervical cancer.

Q: What about the other STD with bumps like genital warts — herpes?

A: That's *genital herpes* and it causes more tears in my office than any other STD, for two reasons. First, when people get an initial outbreak that brings them into the doctor's office, they are usually in significant pain and discomfort. Second, a huge stigma persists associated with a herpes outbreak.

Herpes is a viral disease that lives in nerve cells. There are two types of herpes: herpes simplex virus type I (HSVI) which is most commonly an oral (mouth) or ocular (eye) infection, and herpes simplex virus II (HSVII) which is most commonly found as genital herpes.

It was once thought that you could not spread oral herpes to the genital area, but we now know that is not true. So, beware of the fever blister or mouth sore, since you can spread these to the genital area through oral sex. The good news about spreading oral herpes to the genital area is that the outbreak tends to be much less severe and future outbreaks occur much less often.

Once you are exposed to the herpes virus, there is a 2-10 day incubation period (time from exposure to the outbreak). One of the main problems with herpes is that you can spread the herpes virus and still not know you have ever been infected. In other word, *you are contagious without having a skin outbreak.*

Many people get outbreaks that can range from very mild to very severe. On an initial outbreak, you may first feel like you have the flu. Symptoms may include muscle aches, fever, chills, and swollen glands. Then blisters, or fluid filled sores, may appear in the genital area. There may be a small cluster or a large cluster of blisters.

Q: Is herpes painful?

A: These clusters are often very painful, to the point that people won't urinate because it hurts so badly. The first outbreak can last up to two to three weeks. The blisters often break and weep, but then eventually they crust over toward the end of the outbreak. There are medications that can help relieve the pain and shorten the course of the outbreak. The first outbreak is often the worst. Subsequent outbreaks often have a warning, like burning or itching where the previous outbreak was. This is called a *prodrome* that often develops in the same location as a previous outbreak.

Q: What should I do about it?

A: It is very important to see your health care provider if you think you have an initial herpes outbreak. To diagnose herpes, a culture of the blister fluid at the earliest stage is very helpful, whereas waiting until later in the course of the infection may miss the viral shedding. In other words, if you see your provider and the blisters are mostly crusted over and almost gone, your culture may come back negative, even though you have herpes. However, this does not mean you did not have a herpes infection.

There are new blood tests that have recently become available that are very useful in determining if you have been infected. These blood tests are useful in differentiating between Herpes type 1 and 2. Once you have herpes, you will always have the virus. For your whole life. The good news is that with medication, you can prevent outbreaks and reduce — but not completely eliminate — the chance of spreading the virus.

Sylvia came into the office shortly after she became sexually active, complaining that it hurt when she urinated. She stated that she also felt very irritated on the outside of her vagina. She denied vaginal discharge, but stated that everything hurt very badly and that it was even uncomfortable to sit. The symptoms had just started the day before and she just felt bad all over. To top it off, she even had a fever.

*I asked her to get a urine sample but she said it hurt too bad to go at that time. In the exam room it became apparent she had a severe widespread herpes outbreak. When asked about her sexual partner, she said she had never seen any type of blisters on him. Furthermore, she stated they had both been tested for STDs prior to having sex. He told her he had never had herpes. He had previously had two other sexual partners prior to her and this was her first relationship with intercourse. She was completely confused. How could she have contracted a **herpes infection** if her partner had never had any kind of an outbreak?*

We cultured the widespread lesions to confirm the diagnosis. The next step was to improve her level of comfort using some anesthetic gels and numbing sprays. This gave her some relief.

Then we started the conversation as to how this could happen. She was completely unaware that some people are asymptomatic herpes viral shedders and that her boyfriend could have been infected and never have known. He may be shedding the virus and not having any blister formation. It is very hard to track if he doesn't have outbreaks, but it is a common scenario.

"You probably had intimate contact at a time that he was shedding the virus," I told her. "Your body responded by having the outbreak." I then started her on the antiviral medication twice a day for three days; she also opted to take one pill every day thereafter to try to prevent future outbreaks and to prevent spreading the infection if she had a new sexual partner.

We also discussed the need to pour water on her vulva during urination to help decrease discomfort while emptying her bladder. I also told her to take an analgesic like Motrin® to help the generalized aches and discomforts.

The culture came back positive. To his credit, her partner came into the office as well to try to understand how he could have given her a herpes infection even though he had never had an outbreak. He was equally bewildered. It took a while for him to understand how this could happen. Ultimately, he went to his family physician for a blood test that indicated he had been exposed to the herpes virus at some point. We explained to him that the blood test could tell him if he had been exposed to the virus, but it would not tell him when he was exposed, or if he had an active herpes infection. The concept of being an asymptomatic herpes carrier was very difficult for Sylvia and her partner to grasp, but they came to terms with it. Sylvia's outbreak cleared up in about ten days. She stayed on suppression therapy and hasn't had an outbreak since.

Q: What kind of medicine do I have to take if I have herpes?

A: There are several medication options. Most *suppression medications* are taken once or twice a day. This medication does not get rid of the virus but can help prevent the virus from being active, which decreases viral shedding. It prevents outbreaks and minimizes spreading it to other people.

No one can predict the course that you will follow regarding future outbreaks. Adult women whom I see have come in with an outbreak; when I tell them that they have herpes, they will often remember that they had an initial outbreak years or even decades earlier. Some people who don't take suppression therapy can have outbreaks as often as once a month.

The medication used in the treatment of herpes has been around for a long time with little side effects, and it provides great benefits for treating the disease and preventing outbreaks. If you know you have herpes, it is important to avoid sexual contact during that time so that you minimize the risk of transmitting the infection to a partner.

Q: So I get fever blisters on my mouth. That means I can pass it to my boyfriend's genital area?

A: Yes, you can pass HSV I to the genital area. The most common way for this to happen is through oral sex, or any contact between your saliva and his genitals. Remember, herpes is most contagious prior to the outbreak. So just because you don't have lesions present doesn't mean you are not contagious.

Q: Is that all I have to worry about, or are there other STDs? I think I've heard of "Calamity."

A: Actually, it's *Chlamydia,* the most common bacterial STD, caused by Chlamydia trachomatis. Almost three million people are diagnosed with Chlamydia each year. The incubation period is approximately one to three weeks after exposure. Chlamydia infection can be found in the cervix, which is the most common, or the anus, or the mouth. Therefore the infection can be passed through vaginal, anal or oral sexual activity. More than 75% of women have no symptoms of the infection, and in women who do have symptoms, they can be vague and nonspecific. The most common symptoms are abnormal discharge, burning with urination, pelvic pain or abnormal vaginal bleeding. Men may not know they are infected, as they may have no symptoms either.

I have had a number of patients who come into the office with the complaint of bleeding after sex, which turns out to be due to a Chlamydia lesion. The most common way to diagnose Chlamydia is through a cervical swab that detects the DNA of Chlamydia or through a culture. The treatment for Chlamydia includes various types of antibiotics, *for both people infected*. It is important that all partners get treated and abstain from sexual activity during the treatment period.

A woman often gets re-infected through sexual activity before her partner is treated. Some health care providers may recommend that a repeat test be done in a few months after treatment to be sure that the infection is gone. Untreated, Chlamydia is a major risk factor for infertility and tubal pregnancy, since it can cause scarring in the fallopian tubes. It is recommended that all girls be screened for Chlamydia through the age of 25. I recommend anyone in a new relationship should also be tested.

Kirsten, a 16-year-old patient, came to the office for a routine exam. As usual I recommended that she be tested for STD's. Her exam was normal. However, her lab results were positive for **Chlamydia**. *We gave her a prescription to treat the infection but told her it is critical that her partner also be treated. In fact, they should both abstain from sexual activity until they were both treated.*

I always have patients come back for retesting in about three months, not because the medicine doesn't work but because often both don't get treated or they don't abstain.

Kirsten came back for her 3-month check-up, reporting that she had taken her medication and her boyfriend went to his doctor but was told he didn't need treatment. This concerned me, since the medication is very effective but it simply doesn't work if the partner is not also treated. As expected, she again tested positive for Chlamydia. I re-treated her, stressing that her boyfriend needed treatment or this infection was not going to clear up.

At her follow-up visit Kirsten told me that they had not had sex since they had broken up, but she told him he still needed treatment. I did the test and again it came back positive! I was again concerned. I began to wonder if I had uncovered the first strain of drug resistant Chlamydia or if this was the first time in which the test was simply wrong.

I shared my concerns with Kirsten. She finally admitted that they did have sex. She wasn't sure if he had been treated, but they had used a condom. Most of the time. I spent a lot of time trying to help her understand the risks she is taking by not making sure her partner has had adequate treatment. She nodded with her head, but I'm not sure where her heart was.

Kirsten will return in a few months. Hopefully, this time her test will be negative. In the interim, I will have treated dozens of other Kirstens. Each time, we will have talked about the need to put your health and well being first (including the importance of STD testing), and each time, I have longed to give the Kirstens and their mothers a copy of this as-yet-unwritten book so they don't have to keep coming back.

Q: What about gonorrhea?

A: Gonorrhea is an STD caused by a bacterium called Neisseria gonorrhoea. It is estimated that 700,000 new infections are diagnosed each year. It is spread to the cervix, rectum and mouth through sexual activity. Although, symptoms can be vague with early infection, they can appear in two to 30 days after exposure. The most common symptom is a yellow to green vaginal discharge. Diagnosis is through a culture or DNA testing from a swab. Some offices can do a test called a Gram stain.

There are several antibiotics that can treat a gonorrhea infection. It is extremely important that sexual partners are treated as well. It is often suggested that a test be done to confirm that the infection is cured after treatment. The complications from not treating a gonorrhea condition include infections that travel up the uterus into the tubes and ovaries, arthritis and even infecting the blood, which is very serious.

Q: I've heard of one called trich...

A: That's *trichomoniasis* and it is the most common curable STD in women, affecting 7.4 million women and men per year. The STD is caused by Trichomonas vaginalis, a protozoan parasite that is spread through sexual activity with an infected partner. The symptoms in women include increased green yellow discharge and vaginal itching. The symptoms can be very pronounced.

The most common way trichomoniasis is diagnosed is by examining the discharge under the microscope. A health-care provider can actually see the parasite under the microscope. Metronidazole is the best treatment, usually with a one-dose regimen. A patient and her partner must both be treated in order to prevent reinfection.

Q: What about HIV?

A: Human Immunodeficiency Virus (HIV) is a virus that is spread through intimate sexual contact or contact with infected body fluids such as semen or blood. More than 1,000,000 Americans are infected with HIV. It is thought many other people may be infected and not know it.

The human immunodeficiency virus attacks the cells that help protect your body from infections, causing the immune system to weaken. Often a short time after being infected with the virus, non-specific flu-like symptoms develop such as fever, chills, body aches, and swollen glands. These symptoms often disappear within one to four weeks. More symptoms may not occur again for up to ten years. During the asymptomatic period the immune system of an infected individual can continue to weaken. HIV infection is diagnosed through a blood test that checks for the HIV antibodies. The antibodies generally develop within 6-12 weeks after exposure. There are incidences where the antibodies can take up to six months to develop

Q: Is that the same thing as AIDS?

A: As the disease progresses, patients can have symptoms such as weight loss, chronic yeast infections, night sweats, fevers, fatigue and skin rashes. These are all some of the symptoms most people experience before progressing to Acquired Immunodeficiency Syndrome (AIDS). AIDS is the most advanced stage of HIV infection.

Early detection of the infection is important so that an infected person can be placed on medications to help prevent the infection from progressing to AIDS. Remember, *HIV is not spread through casual contact, but through semen or blood.* Condoms are your best protection, as well as limiting the number of sexual partners. Sharing of needles should definitely be avoided, as the virus can easily spread through used syringes and needles.

Q: Are there any other STDs I should know about?

A: Syphilis is an STD caused by a bacterium named Treponema pallidum. Syphilis is spread through contact with an infected skin sore called a chancre — a painless sore that lasts 3-6 weeks after its appearance. The chancre usually appears 10-90 days after exposure, the average being 21 days.

This is called primary syphilis. If it is treated at this point, there are usually no permanent problems. The treatment for primary syphilis is an antibiotic injection. The most common sign of secondary syphilis is generally a rash that does not itch, but will also go away without treatment. If treatment is not instituted at this stage it will progress to late stage or tertiary syphilis. This form of syphilis is very dangerous, causing damage to the brain, leading to internal injuries, problems with muscle coordination, blindness, dementia and even death.

And don't forget about *hepatitis*, which is an inflammation of the liver. There are several viruses that can cause hepatitis, including Hepatitis B and C. Hepatitis can be transmitted in several ways including through sexual activity, blood, and bodily fluids. The most common strain to spread though sexual activity is Hepatitis B. The good news is that now children are required to receive a Hepatitis B vaccine at birth. If you feel you are at risk for hepatitis you should have blood tests to evaluate for it. Other important risks for hepatitis are tattooing and piercing using nonsterile needles, which have led to an increase in the number of Hepatitis C cases. So if you have had piercing or a new tattoo, it is reasonable to be tested.

Q: Should I have an STD check with every well woman exam?

A: The answer is yes, yes, yes! I always recommend that young women should be tested with their annual exam. The formal recommendation is testing for all sexually active women through age 25. Many of the infections such as chlamydia have no symptoms. Untreated it can cause damage to your uterus, tubes and ovaries, so it is important to be tested. Even for women who are over 25 in new relationships, I suggest testing.

The chlamydia and gonorrhea tests are done while you are having your Pap test and, of course, the Pap screens for HPV. The other recommended tests are done through blood. The tests I recommend are for HIV, Syphilis, and hepatitis in certain situations. Hepatitis testing should be done especially for patients with multiple sexual partners or ones with tattoos and/or piercings. Knowing that you do not have an STD can be very reassuring.

Q: Are there symptoms I should look for as a sign I have an STD?

A: Many STDs do not cause symptoms, but some do. It is important, whenever you have a symptom that concerns you, to see your health care professional. Some of the most common symptoms that bring people to the doctor's office are usually bumps in the vaginal area. Remember, not all bumps are STDs, but bumps are definitely a reason to be seen. The most important bumps are blisters — painful, ulcerated or wart looking bumps.

The other symptoms commonly seen are irregular vaginal bleeding or pain with intercourse. Vaginal discharge is also a common symptom seen in association with STDs, but *remember vaginal discharge can and is often a normal thing.* You should pay attention to discharge in larger than normal amounts, discharge that is yellow to green colored, or discharge that itches or has an odor.

Q: Can I get an STD from making out but not having intercourse?

A: You definitely can get STDs without have intercourse. Oral sex is a common way STDs are transmitted. Certain STDs can be passed through intimate touching of penis or vulva. For example, HPV and herpes virus can be passed from skin to skin contact. The best way to prevent STDs is through no intimate contact. However, if you are having any intimate contact, be tested for infections. ***Always practice safe sex.***

Q: Are there signs or symptoms I should look for in my boyfriend that indicate he may be infected with an STD?

A: Many STDs will not have any visible signs or symptoms. For men especially, infections such as Chlamydia, HPV and often herpes are completely asymptomatic. On rare occasions they can have discharge from the penis or burning with urination. However if you see any growths or ulcerations, *ask questions.* And stay away from intimate contact until you both have been tested.

Q: How concerned should I be if my Pap smear is abnormal?

A: That depends on the results. If you have abnormal cells, see if they can do an HPV test. The results of the HPV test can help determine how important the abnormality is. If you are positive for high risk type HPV you need to do what your health care professional recommends in a timely manner. You should not panic, but do not wait months to follow up. Most abnormal Pap smears can be taken care of easily in the office by your health care provider.

Q: I have an abnormal Pap smear and was told I need a colposcopy. How is this done?

A: A colposcopy is a test done in the event of an abnormal Pap test. The test enables a health care professional to look at the cervix under magnification and determine if there are abnormal areas on the cervix that need to be "biopsied." An acidic liquid (no worries, it's only vinegar) is applied to the cervix, making the abnormality more visible. If biopsies are needed they will take a pinch of the tissue to send to the lab for testing. The most noticeable pain is a cramping sensation.

Some people use a spray that numbs the cervix, but it is unclear how much of a difference this makes. To decrease pain, we generally tell patients to take ibuprofen prior to the procedure.

The test is done in the office. In fact, most women are able to leave the office right away. The *colposcopy test* is an important test, for it will help tell how abnormal the cells on the Pap test are and what the risk is for cervical cancer.

Q: I think I may have been exposed to a sexually transmitted infection. Where can I get tested and will I have to tell my parents?

A: Anytime you think you have been exposed to an STD you need to be tested so that it can be treated as soon as possible. Planned Parenthood will do screening and exams without parent notification unless local legislation says otherwise. In general, you can probably test without your parent finding out.

Even though it seems very hard for some teens to consider talking to their parents about sexual activity, I still encourage a patient to do so—usually. The sense I get from the patient about their relationship will guide this decision. Often I will see both the patient and parent to help facilitate this discussion. I will never tell a parent without permission from the daughter unless I am forced to by law. I also encourage parents to allow girls to have a patient-healthcare relationship where they can confide in the provider without concerns of the parents finding out information.

Q: How effective are condoms in preventing STDs?

A: Condom use will definitely not completely protect you from all STD exposures. But, other than abstinence, it is your best protection, especially against HIV. They are quite effective against gonorrhea and Chlamydia. Some infections, like herpes or HPV, are spread through intimate contact instead of only through body fluids and, therefore, condoms may not completely protect you. Remember, other than abstinence, condoms will offer the best protection against STDs.

Q: What is PID?

A: Pelvic inflammatory disease (PID) is an infection of the upper genital tract. The uterus, fallopian tubes and/or ovaries are involved. As many as one million women are affected every year. Indeed, it is the number one preventable cause of female infertility. As many as 100 women will die each year from PID. Untreated Gonorrhea and Chlamydia are often the primary cause. PID symptoms can be sudden and severe. Symptoms include fever, vaginal discharge, painful urination, painful intercourse, irregular vaginal bleeding and abdominal pain.

If you think that you have PID, it is extremely important to see a health care provider as soon as possible since early treatment can reduce long term damage to the genital tract. Treatment of early infection includes oral antibiotics. More advanced cases of PID can require hospitalization and intravenous antibiotics. Diagnostic tests include evaluating for gonorrhea, chlyamidia, HIV and syphilis. A pelvic ultrasound may have to be done if it is suspected that an abscess (pus filled area) may be present in the tubes or ovaries.

MOM QUESTIONS

Here are some mother's questions related to STDs and vaginal health. Listen in, daughters, since they may relate to you.

Q: I had abnormal Pap smears as a young woman. Now my daughter has abnormal Pap tests. Does that mean I passed this to her?

A: No, you did not pass it on to her. HPV is responsible for most abnormal Pap tests, which is generally transmitted through intimate or sexual contact. Since HPV tests can be done during a Pap test, it is easy to determine if your daughter has been exposed to HPV. There is no evidence that I am aware of that shows a genetic predisposition to cervical abnormalities.

Q: My daughter was diagnosed with genital herpes and swears that she has not had sex. Should I believe her?

A: It depends how you define sex. If you only define it as intercourse, you can believe her. However, there is probably some pretty intimate contact if your child was diagnosed with genital herpes. It is important to explore with her what kinds of sexual activity she is having. (This will be discussed in Chapter 4 on sexuality and relationships).

Q: My daughter went for a check up and they tested her for STDs. Why would they do this if they don't suspect her of having an infection?

A: The standard of care is to test women for sexually transmitted diseases at their annual exam through the age of 26. I encourage all of my young patients to be tested since so many STDs have no signs or symptoms. Early detection of an infection can prevent some of the problems that can occur with an undiagnosed and untreated infection.

Q: I had an STD when I was younger. Should I tell my daughter about my sexual past?

A: This is a difficult question and I usually recommend you be very careful before bringing something like this up to discuss. It would be wise to bring this up only if you think it may help your daughter to understand your point of view. It may help her understand why you seem "overprotective" or if she views you as being "too strict" in your views about sex. When you tell your daughter this you will want to do it at a time when you have plenty of opportunity to explain what happened and you don't feel rushed. You will want to tell her how this affected your life and any sex you subsequently had after you acquired the disease. You will want to tell her how you may have felt "stigmatized" and how you learned to deal with those feelings. If your daughter understands that what happened to you affected you so deeply that you do not want her to have the same negative experience, she will understand that you care for her and love her. She may be able to learn from your mistakes in the past. As a general guideline, I do not advise bringing up your past unless it is in your daughter's best interest.

TABLE TALK

Table Talk Conversations on STDs. (Jerrilyn, 17-year-old girl, talking to her mom about a possible exposure to an STD and the need to be tested; Mom [Miranda] is cooking dinner; no one else is home and the house is quiet)

Jerrilyn: Mom I have to tell you something and I don't want you to freak out.

Miranda (stops cooking and sits down at the table with her daughter): Okay, tell me what is up?

Jerrilyn: I am worried that I have caught something because I found these bumps down there (pointing to the vaginal area) and they really hurt.

Miranda: What do you think they are?

Jerrilyn: Maybe it is herpes?

Miranda: Herpes? Have you done something that would cause you to get herpes?

Jerrilyn: Well, I haven't had sex.

Miranda: If you haven't had sex, what do you think these are?

Jerrilyn: I don't know

Miranda: I want to help you, which means I need you to be really honest with me about any kind of intimate contact that you have had.

Jerrilyn: Well, Jimmy (boyfriend of one month) and I have done some making out.

Miranda: (calmly): Making out? Which means you have only kissed?

Jerrilyn: Well, a little more than that.

Miranda: How much more?

Jerrilyn: Well, we've done a fair bit of touching.

Miranda: Just touching ...

Jerrilynn: Well, we had oral sex once, but we have not had sex.

Miranda: So you don't think oral sex is sex?

Jerrilynn: Not exactly, not really. But what do I need to do now?

Miranda: Lets go have you tested for STD and continue this talk once we see what is going on.

Conversation Starters

For moms:

1. Do they teach you about sexually transmitted diseases in school?

2. The new vaccine for cervical cancer is wonderful. I think you should get it.

3. I read an article in the newspaper that sexually transmitted infections can be passed through oral sex. I don't think I knew that. Did you?

For daughters:

1. You wouldn't believe what we are talking about in health class. Did they teach you about sexually transmitted infections when you were in school?

2. Why do I need to get the vaccine for HPV if I am not sexually active?

3. Mom, my friend's mom told her that if she became sexually active she would buy her condoms to protect her against STDs. What do you think about that?

CHAPTER **4**

"I Wanna Know"

SEXUALITY AND RELATIONSHIPS

W omen's health care providers often find that adolescent girls have little understanding of how their bodies function or the risks involved when they become sexually active. Recent studies repeatedly demonstrate that the average adolescent has sexual intercourse for the first time at 15 years of age. Teenage pregnancy rates are higher in the United States than other post-industrial countries, and they are twice as high as the rates in both Canada and England. Millions of teens are also diagnosed with sexually transmitted infections every year. When teen girls are asked if they considered the consequences of unprotected sexual intercourse, the vast majority usually replies "no."

Why are our adolescents so prone to these generally unintended yet quite preventable consequences of early sexual activity? **The primary reason is that** teenage girls mature physically sooner than they mature cognitively. The average age of menstruation in the United States is 11 years. In contrast, a girl's prefrontal cortex — the part of the brain that is responsible for organizing thought, understanding consequences, and interpreting emotions — is not fully developed until she is well into her twenties. In other words, while the teen girl's body is telling her to be sexually active, her brain is having a difficult time understanding the bigger picture.

Teen girls need help understanding how their sexuality is developing and how to make informed decisions that will affect their physical health and emotional well-being. By not giving our daughters accurate, truthful information and by not taking advantage of opportunities for frank discussion, we *fail* to prepare them. We *fail* to equip them to deal with the health and sexual issues that they face at an early age. As the statistics show, we are falling short in educating our adolescent girls about the consequences of sexual activity and in teaching them how they can and should protect themselves.

> *One day, I was seeing patients in the office when my oldest daughter called me from the school cafeteria to ask me to settle a dispute among her friends (most of whom I knew well and whose voices I could hear in the background.) The question was "do you lose your virginity with oral sex?" Some of her friends were saying that oral sex was "completely safe" and that it really was "no big deal."*

> *After I got over the initial shock that my 7th grader had been discussing the subject of a boy's penis in a girl's mouth, I took a deep breath and began to explore this topic with my daughter. I learned a few things from our talk. First, girls — even at that young age — talk about sex with their friends, and what they say is not necessarily accurate. Second, my daughter felt that she could ask me a potentially jarring question, because she and her friends wanted information from a trustworthy and knowledgeable source. Apparently I qualified. Third, my daughter felt pressure from her friends to regard oral sex as safe and acceptable behavior, and*

she wanted my support for her contrary view. She felt that she needed my help to stand up to this pressure, and I was glad to be there for her. I was reminded of how important it is to know your daughter's peer group.

Outside education is not enough; education is most effective when it takes place in the context of a trusted relationship. For instance, take a look at popular school-based substance abuse prevention programs: character-based (e.g., "Just Say No"), fear-based (e.g., "Scared Straight"), information-based (e.g., "This is Your Brain on Drugs), intelligence-based (e.g., "Smart People Don't Do Drugs"). Students who participated in the prevention programs were found to use drugs *at earlier ages,* and *more frequently* than students who had not participated at all. Participation in the program had a negative, rather than positive, effect across the board, with one exception: those that took place in the context of strong social bonding, or strong school-family interactions. A strong resiliency effect was noted for those programs presented *in the context of a caring adult.*

Also, studies have shown that parent-child closeness in discussing sexuality leads to the initiation of sexual activity at an *older and more mature age,* with a *lower frequency of risky behaviors,* such as ignoring safe sex practices. Adolescent girls report the desire to learn about sex and healthy living from their mother, and a mother remains the one person who can best influence the information that her adolescent girl receives.

Consequently, we mothers must take the opportunity—indeed, the obligation—to educate our daughters about sex seriously, because teaching our daughters about sex and keeping themselves safe is as important as teaching them to tie their shoes. Simply telling our daughters that we are there for them if they have any questions is NOT enough. We must step up to the plate and bring the subject up, talk to them, take them out for coffee. We must share our ideas about sexual health, relationships and healthy living, just as we do about academic plans.

As we've said before, health care providers often see young women *after* problems occur—problems that might have been avoided if the adolescents had received adequate sex education. Failure to equip our daughters with detailed, adequate and accurate information about sexuality that recognizes both their physical maturity and emotional immaturity can have life-long consequences. Of concern are not only such consequences as teenage pregnancy, abortion, and STDs, but also one which seldom gets acknowledged: the difficulty in forming healthy adult sexual relationships in their future.

We would like to highlight one more point before moving on to Q&A's. We believe sex is *"sacro."* *Sacro sex* is the concept that sexuality is a sacred union. It means you value, respect, and cherish the relationship. *Sacro sex* is patient, it perseveres, it maintains high standards. Since we believe it's important for both moms and daughters to understand the centrality of *sacro sex*, we'll make sure to work it to the Q&A for mothers as well as daughters.

DAUGHTER QUESTIONS

Probably the questions that generate the most emotion have to do with sexuality and relationships. They are also the hardest for moms and daughters to broach. We'll start with questions from you, girls and daughters, but your moms will definitely want to listen in.

Q: What is the best age to begin dating?

A: This is a difficult question, because with my own daughters I encouraged school activities and jobs after school. They didn't have time to date except for the Prom, Homecoming and Cotillion. Every girl is so individual. Some are really into sports and others really want social activities or satisfy their passion with school events.

I will offer my best overall feelings to your question, though, because I want the best for you. I think sixteen is a good age to begin dating. Before the age of sixteen dating is unnecessary because there are so many ways you can get together and enjoy each other within a group. Teenager's frontal cortexes are not fully developed until the age of nineteen (and sometimes it takes longer); therefore, they often react impulsively and may not be rational. Love is a drug. It actually produces hormones that make us blind to real facts about the other person.

At the age of sixteen you have so much ahead of you, that I think it is unwise to think that this is the "one and only." Boys at sixteen may like or even love you, but mostly they are curious and will want to experiment sexually. No matter what they say, you most likely will not be the love of their life. Boys may love the way you make them feel, but they are inexperienced and often can not separate that love from the loving you part. If you date at sixteen, remember that sexual intercourse and oral sex are *sacro*. Save that part for someone when you are older and wiser and can give that part of your body to someone because you are ready and mature enough to handle a relationship. Wait until you know for sure who you are and where you want to go in your life.

Many times, girls date and do things they don't want to do, because they feel pressured, and they feel like they *need* a boyfriend. Don't let yourself fall into that trap. You need good friends, and a mom you can talk to who is there to guide you and help you become the best you can be. I want that for you too!!!!

Q: My boyfriend keeps pressuring me to have sex with him, but I'm not ready yet. How can I tell him without ruining our relationship?

A: I am more concerned that you will ruin any possible relationship if you *don't* tell him that you are not ready. Your boyfriend may want sex because he thinks that is what he should do, if he is a "real guy." Many times, boys pressure girls for sex just to "fit in." Your boyfriend may be curious about sex, but trying to fit in and being curious are not good enough reasons to have sex. He may have no idea what sex is and what it will mean. If you have sex with him, the feelings he feels afterward may make him feel shameful, or guilty. He may break up with you anyway, and then not only are you dealing with a ruined relationship, but also feelings of guilt or shame that you gave a part of yourself away that you can never have back.

Your sexuality and intimacy belong to you to keep or give away. You have to be emotionally mature (which usually doesn't happen until after the age of eighteen) and able to talk about sexuality. You have to be comfortable with the idea of possibly getting pregnant or contracting a sexually transmitted disease. Are you able to handle either of these consequences right now? If you are not, it is not time for you to have sex. It would be wiser to tell your boyfriend that you really care for him, but you are not ready for accepting possible consequences. Tell him that you feel so close to him that you do not want to do anything that could possibly ruin the relationship. What I hear in this question is that you are not ready to have sex, and you would be wise to explore options of feeling close to your boyfriend in ways other than sex.

The important points, I believe, are focusing on maturity and knowing when "you're ready," because this is not only a huge step in a relationship but also individually. It is also important to emphasize that there are alternatives to jumping into bed together.

> *Before I got married I was dating a boy who lived about a two-hour-drive from me. I was in college and not able to drive (no car), and he was in the same situation. We found some very creative ways to keep in touch. (There was no Internet nor any other form of instant communication). We kept a special jar into which we placed little notes as we thought about each other all week. I would add strips of paper that mentioned different places we could be together when next we saw each other, or little love notes of how I was thinking of him during the week. Then we would mail the jars (I think they were plastic peanut butter jars) to each other at the end of the week. We both loved it! It was so neat to be able to read what he had written, ideas he had generated. We were best friends, and we loved each other. We knew we didn't want to sacrifice the relationship by having sex too soon.*

Get creative with your own ways of expressing love without sex. Remember, in the end what is important is that you understand and really care about what is best for the two of you.

Q: I want to wait until marriage to have sex, but sometimes I feel like I am going to say yes. Is this a common feeling?

A: Yes, this is a very common feeling. Many girls have sex because they don't know another way to express love and affection for their boyfriend. Many girls have sex because they want to fit in, or their friends are having it, or out of curiosity. We all are susceptible to our surroundings.

If you want to wait until marriage to have sex, surround yourself with friends who feel like you do. There is power and strength in hanging out with like-minded friends. You can support each other, and that helps so much with resisting behaviors that you do not feel are in your best interest.

I also think it is important to talk to your boyfriend about how you feel. If he respects you, and he wants what is best for you (and for the two of you as a couple), he will honor your wishes. Sex is something that is beautiful when shared in a monogamous, stable relationship. It is only part of a relationship. It is not just an action. It is a way of expressing deep love and affection in a relationship. I have seen it make a relationship better, and I have also seen it ruin relationships.

Engaging in sex before you have a strong committed relationship is the quickest way to kill a relationship. When a woman wants to wait for marriage and she goes against her own beliefs and wishes, she ends up resentful at the man who took that belief or desire away. Make your own decisions about your own body, and stay true to them!! You do have total control over your own body, though, and if this is your wish you can make it happen!

Q: What is masturbation?

A: Masturbation is when you touch yourself, stimulating yourself to make yourself "feel good." It is completely normal. Most girls masturbate from the age of three to four until they are about seven. Masturbation is not dirty or wrong and it is not considered having sex. Many religions are not comfortable with masturbation, though it is actually a normal, healthy human activity that can relieve stress and calm people. It is not okay to masturbate in public. When my daughters were small and touched their private parts, I would suggest that if they wanted to engage in that activity they do it in the privacy of their bedroom. Teenagers as well as adults should follow this advice to engage in masturbation during their private times.

Q: Sometimes I feel sexually curious, or feel just plain "horny."
Does this make me weird?

A: Girls are just as curious as boys about sexuality, their developing bodies, and physical sensations. In fact, as we noted earlier, there are biological reasons for increased female libido. Curiosity is normal; so is feeling aroused. In fact, it is our hope that this book will spark conversations with your mother about that. After 25 years of working with developing girls, we are convinced more than ever that understanding how your body works is important, as is understanding the *sacro* nature of sex.

Q: Does making out with a girl one time mean I am a lesbian?

A: No, it does not make you a lesbian. It does suggest that you are curious and trying to see where you fit. If you feel more confused after making out with a girl one time and you enjoyed it more than kissing a boy or holding his hand it could possibly mean you have some tendencies toward lesbian behavior. Most lesbian women I have spoken with tell me they have always preferred women and thought it repulsive to consider being as close to a boy. Remember, you can still contract an STD from another girl.

Q: Do you lose your virginity with oral sex?

A: No, you do not lose your virginity, but you are engaging in sex. Virginity means that a penis has never entered into the vagina. The hymen membrane may be intact. You cannot rupture the hymen with oral sex; however, you can get many nasty diseases with oral sex. We do not recommend it until after the age of eighteen and after you have been friends with this special person for at least one year. Unfortunately we know that boyfriends and girlfriends will tell us they love us to get a personal need met. Be warned. You are sacro—divine. Do what is best for your body and heart.

Q: If I've had sex and he acts differently, what do I do?

A: First of all let me say I am sorry. This is a question I hear frequently and I understand how hurt and confused you probably feel.

He told you he loved you, and you had sex. Now you realize neither of you were ready, and he deals with it by withdrawing and walking away, and you cling more and call him but he basically isn't interested.

I would suggest you talk to him. Explain to him how you feel. Try not to blame him. Take responsibility for your action and forgive yourself. I also suggest you confide in your mom and explain how you feel. Talk with your mom about what you were thinking would happen. Did you expect him to like you more? Did you have sex because you thought you had to?

All of these things will be important for you to share with your mom. She will want to take you for a check-up to be sure that you are okay and haven't been exposed to a sexually transmitted disease. This is very important. We all live and learn, so don't be too hard on yourself, but do use it as a lesson to yourself of what not to do in the next relationship.

Q: What should I do if my parents don't like my boyfriend?

A: Congratulations! The fact that you are asking this question tells me that what your parents think is important to you, and that says a lot about you. Most parents don't like boyfriends if they see certain characteristics. They don't like impolite boys, risk taking behavior, anger outbursts, or domestic violence. They worry if the boy doesn't like his own parents, and mostly they don't like boys who are disrespectful of their daughter (that's you).

Now, that being said, let me explain it this way. Look how wise you are compared to your ten- or eight-year-old brother or sister. Would you worry for them? Of course you would. Your parents feel the same in regards to you. They are much older and experienced. A lot has changed over the years, but relationships have not for the most part. Your mom and dad have lived a lot. Listen to them, talk to them, and explain what you appreciate about your boyfriend. If he is a worthy boyfriend he will try to work with your parents. If he is not a keeper, he will tear up your driveway with his car when he gets mad at your parents. In that case you can do better.

TABLE TALK

Boyfriend Issues. Here is a suggestion of how to start a discussion about your boyfriend with your mom and dad. You may feel comfortable starting out by talking with your mother alone. Many times, girls tell me it is intimidating to talk to both mom and dad at the same time. I suggest you "set the table," and by now you know that means to choose a time when you are not rushed. Maybe you could talk over a cup of hot tea or a soft drink? When you talk to your mom, you want to make sure you are open and not feeling angry before the conversation even begins. If you are angry this is not a conversation to discuss something. Instead it becomes a "Let me convince you lecture" that neither you nor mom would enjoy. Let's pretend your name is Elena.

Elena: Mom, can we plan some time to talk?

Mom: I would love that... when?

Elena: How about in 15 minutes.

Mom: Sounds great, let's meet at the kitchen table.

(15 minutes go by...........).

Elena: Thanks for taking the time to talk to me, Mom. I need to talk to you about Gary, my boyfriend.

Mom: Oh, is something wrong?

Elena: Well, sorta... not really, I don't know.

Mom: What's going on, Elena?

Elena: I just wish you liked him. It makes me feel bad that you and Daddy don't. I feel like I am being sneaky when I am with him, and not honest to you or to Gary.

Mom: I am sorry, Honey. That wasn't my or your father's intention. We don't really know Gary. I feel like you "hide" him and that makes me feel like you are ashamed of him. I then start to worry that he isn't good to you.

Elena: I feel like it is a cycle. I think you don't like him, so I don't invite him to be around you, and now I just feel like you don't like him.

Mom: I don't know him, Elena. I cannot say if I like him until I am involved more with him.

Elena: Well... I love you and Daddy. It makes it hard to date or care for someone you both don't seem to like.

Mom: Why don't you invite Gary over for dinner this week? That way, maybe we can learn a little bit more about him, and help guide you in a way that won't feel like we don't like him. If he treats you well... and he understands that your education comes first along with all of your own passions... then I think I will like him.

Elena: Thanks, Mom. I will invite him over this week. Is there a day that works best for you? (If mom is inviting him for dinner, make sure it is a date that works for her. That is showing respect for your mother's time and effort).

Mom: I think a Tuesday or a Thursday would work for us. That way, after dinner you will still have time to work on your projects, and I can get my paper work done before bedtime.

Elena: Thanks so much, Mom... you are the best!!!

Mom: I love you, Elena. I look forward to getting to know Gary.

Q: Does sexual intercourse have to hurt the first time?

A: Yes, the first time it is usually uncomfortable. There are several reasons it usually hurts. The first has to do with anatomy. The vagina does stretch, but the first time it is usually very tight. Lubrication helps the penis enter, but the first time most girls are nervous and they don't lubricate as well. Most girls are having sex with a boy who doesn't really know how to make love, either, so he goes too fast and it is not very satisfying.

Love-making feels better when it is in a committed relationship. There is more caring for each other, and the couple moves slower, understanding this will make the experience more pleasurable. When you love someone you trust them fully, and this makes you more relaxed and the muscles aren't as tight. When you are more mature and in a committed, loving relationship, sexual intercourse makes the relationship even more committed and loving. Without the relationship, sexual intercourse leaves the woman feeling used, cold and alone. No matter what anyone says about "friends with benefits," the benefits are only for the boy (and usually not him either). A woman never gains anything from having casual sex—except a nice big STD.

Q: My best friend talks about being sexual all the time, what should I do?

A: If she isn't a really good friend ignore her and walk away. If you are fairly close and you are worried about her, tell her so. Many times girls talk about having sex if they feel that it will make them more popular. She may be trying to fit in or get more attention. She could be crying for help, so someone will be concerned and ask her what's going on. Usually girls who do this are insecure and trying to rebel or appear more attractive. It is not emotionally healthy, and if everyone ignores her she will most likely come up with a new conversation to appear hip. Usually any girl who has to announce her sexuality is doing so to get a reaction. She may have severe body image problems. You may just want to ask her in a manner like the conversation below:

TABLE TALK

Table Talk Conversation with Friend about Sexuality.

Your friend: (... Something about herself being sexual ....)

Your response: Hey, are you okay?

Your friend: Yeah, why are you asking me that?

Your response: Well, you talk a lot about sex lately, and I am concerned (or worried about you), because you used to never do that.

Your friend: (Starts getting tears in her eyes, and maybe tells you what is really going on, or she may say, "Yeah, I am fine". Don't be surprised if she calls you later, though, and tells you the truth about something that is going on.)

Q: What is an orgasm, and will I have one when I have sex?

A: An orgasm is a climax, or when you reach the peak of your sexual excitement. It is a contraction of muscles within the vagina and it feels like a release of tension. It is very common to feel like you are secreting a fluid and although it is not like an ejaculation, you do secrete more fluid at this time. It feels absolutely wonderful, and it is a release of tension built up during the sex act. Most girls do not experience an orgasm the first time they have sex, or they may have one while masturbating but not be able to have one during intercourse. Sometimes, it seems that the more you try to have one the less chance you will have one. I know many grown women who have never had an orgasm. Most of sex occurs in the mind, and this is certainly true of orgasm.

It is a normal part of sex and it is important that you learn about your own body so you understand what parts of the genitals and your entire body bring you pleasure before you expect anyone else to understand how to please you. Some women make a noise when they orgasm and some do not. Most movies show women screaming and doing all kinds of things during an orgasm. You may feel like screaming, moaning, jumping, the list is endless. Or, you may feel like holding your partner tighter and not saying anything. There is no right or wrong way to have an orgasm.

You do not have to have an orgasm to become pregnant, and having an orgasm in and of itself will not make you pregnant. You can get pregnant with or without an orgasm.

Q: I have a friend who said she is a "secondary virgin." What is that, and can I become one?

A: Secondary virgins confuse me, but I understand why girls want to be called that. What that means is that a girl has had sex for what she feels is the wrong reason, or against her religious beliefs. She feels like she reflects and repents it, and then says to herself and her friends or family, "From this day forward I will not have sex with anyone until I get married to them."

It is a big decision, and most girls who make it have a difficult time keeping that sort of promise. They can do it though, if it is really important to them and if they have a loving supportive family and friends. You don't need to be a secondary virgin unless you have already had sex and believe it was a poor choice.

I really encourage mothers and daughters to talk openly about this sort of topic. Moms can really help if they don't judge their daughters but try to give them support and guidance. As you know, I do not believe any girl should have sex before the age of eighteen. I think it is important that you have a clear understanding of yourself and your goals and education. If you focus on your passions in life and understand what it is you want, you will be more prepared to make better decisions about sexuality in the future. I have never seen a girl who had sex before the age of eighteen who would not have waited until she was more mature if she was given a second chance. You have to consider that an important statement. I see and talk to many girls all over the country.

Q: My best friend told me her boyfriend went to "second base" with her. She wanted to know how to stop.

A: You must be a good friend if your friend asked you such a vulnerable question. I think that is great, and I will trust you will give her this advice and be loyal to her. I don't know how old your friend is, but if she is under eighteen years old second base is not a good idea. My idea of second base is fondling of the breasts and genitals. That is like setting fire to one dry branch in a forest of dry trees. Things are going to keep going further and she may not be able to say "No."

Encourage your friend to talk to her boyfriend. She needs to tell him she has goals and passions in her own life. She should tell him that she really likes him and respects him, and wants to stay close to him. If she explains that things could get out of control and they would both lose the friendship if they did, he will listen. Your friend should tell him this at a time they are doing something like walking around in the mall or eating lunch. It should be said at a time when they are just together and enjoying each other's company. It cannot be said in the heat of the moment, as he may feel rejected, or angry, and this will hurt your friend.

When I was a girl I was asked out by a boy I was crazy about. I was so happy; I had wanted to date him forever. He took me out and started touching under my shirt, my breasts, opened my pants. I was so embarrassed; I didn't know how to tell him to stop. Finally I had to scream it, or I would not have had the courage to say it. Needless to say, he dropped me off and we never spoke again. When I think back to that time I still feel badly. I wish I would have thought to talk to him beforehand; it could have gone so much better.

Boys are curious. They want to touch girls and see their bodies. Of course, girls are curious too and may want to do the same things to boys. Girls have to remember that it is not our job to please boys. It is our job to take care of and respect ourselves. We should expect boys to respect us, but if we don't have clear boundaries and the confidence to define those boundaries then unfortunately boys won't either.

Q: *What is a "friend with benefits?"*

A: Good question. This is a term that became popular about five years ago. It is a term that is used by girls mostly, and it means you have a friend with whom you also have sex. It is usually not a good idea, because no matter how we may act or talk, someone usually gets hurt in this relationship. It is mostly for people who don't want to commit to actually having someone that they are faithful with, and so they "hang out" with their best friend and also have sex. This friend can be someone the girl or boy respects but it is usually not. After all, if you really respected the person why would you get involved in doing such an intimate act (sharing your body) but not committing to them?

Most girls who engage in this arrangement end up being hurt and unhappy. If you want to have sex with someone, do your homework and make sure it is someone worthwhile; someone who has your best interests at heart. Why would you want to share something sacred like your body, with someone who used you for sex because there wasn't something better around?

Q: What is date rape?

A: Date rape is when you are out with someone and sex is forced on you. You do not consent to it, and in fact may say "no," but the person you are with assaults you anyway. This can involve force or drugs given to you so that you will not fight off your attacker. Many times date rape happens when it was not intended to happen. Two people can be out on a date and are fondling each other and kissing each other, but then things go too far. When the girl realizes she does not want to have intercourse and tries to call it off the boy is already in the act of starting sexual intercourse. These two people usually do not have a well developed relationship yet and cannot talk about sexuality openly. That is a dangerous situation, and usually goes from bad to worse.

Sex is sacred, and it should always be done between two consenting adults who are mature enough to have a longstanding, openly communicative relationship. Sexual intercourse is a beautiful act to express love between two mature adults, but it can also be a very cruel way to express hatred and power in the case of rape.

Q: What should I do if I am the victim of rape?

A: If you are the victim of rape, the first thing I will tell you is that it is not your fault. Never, no how, no matter what the perpetrator says. It doesn't matter if he tells you that you teased him, or led him on, or whatever other sick thing he says. *"No" means "No."* It always has and always will!

What you must do now is not panic. Tell someone immediately. I recommend your mom, best friend, or both. You will need someone to take you to a hospital emergency room. Do not shower, and do not change your clothes, no matter how much you want to. The ER staff will want to look for evidence of semen, and the only way they can do that is if you haven't washed or changed your clothes. They will want to check your vaginal area and possibly your rectum. They will want to test for STD and they most likely will do a blood test. It will be scary and you will feel cold. Make sure someone brings a warm jacket for you, and possibly a blanket.

You need to do this for several reasons. The first is to assure that you are okay, and if there is a problem you can get treatment immediately. The second is to make sure there is evidence so the authorities can hold whoever did this accountable. Lastly, you are doing it for every woman. We now know that a rapist doesn't rape just one person. If he gets away with it after hurting you, he will usually do it again, and again to someone else. You are actually helping to save other women from going through what you experienced. Sex offenders (that's the person who raped you) are deeply disturbed people with a serious degree of mental illness. They don't rape women for the way the women look or what they said. They rape because they are mentally sick and they think they will not get caught.

Q: My friends don't really talk about rape, or even being molested. Am I the only one?

A: Sexual harassment is unwelcome and intrusive attention of a sexual nature that may involve verbal, visual, or physical conduct. Child sexual molestation refers to sexual abuse of a child by an adult, or some other person significantly older or in a position of power or control over the child, where the child is used for sexual stimulation of another person.

It is said that two out of four women in the United States are raped, molested or sexually harassed by the age of 25 years. This sounds unbelievable, until you start talking to your friends and your mom's friends. I had a Pajama Party for my adult friends one evening. We started talking about this topic. There were six of us there. Out of the six of us, four of us fit the category of having been sexually harassed or molested by the age of 25 years. How does that happen? Well, for one thing, we didn't feel empowered to say "No." We didn't feel empowered to tell someone or scream. I now work in a Weight Loss Clinic. Guess what I found out? Yep, that's right. Many women who are severely obese have been raped or molested as small children. They gain weight as a protection from men. They have no idea why they cannot keep the weight off. They have hidden the rape deep into their mind.

If you are ever molested, raped, or sexually harassed, tell someone. That is the first giant step. If you can do that, everything will get better. Who should you tell? Tell your mom. If she doesn't believe you, tell your mom's best friend, your dad, whomever you trust. You did not deserve it. It wasn't your fault.

Q: How does someone drug me to have sex with me?

A: The date rape drug most commonly used is called Rohypnol. It is commonly referred to as "roofies." The chemical name is flunitrazepam and it is a cousin to a drug called diazepam (better known as Valium®). It makes whoever takes it feel dopey and lethargic. The rapist usually puts it in your drink; therefore, you should be careful what you drink and whom you are with at a party. It's not just boys who may slip the drug in your drink; sometimes a girl who doesn't think you are so neat will slip it in your drink to watch you get drugged. There are several other date rape drugs, but the problem isn't the drug, it is what kind of a "psycho" uses them. Here is the main message: know where you are going and with whom you are going. If you go in a group, watch out for your friends. It's also a good idea that an adult (like your parent) knows where you are going and with whom.

Q: My best friend was sexually abused. How can I help her?

A: The best way to help a friend who has been sexually abused is to realize that being a good listener is the greatest gift you can give her. You will not be able to solve her problems though, and you should never try to handle it on your own. Encourage your friend to talk with her mom (if she hasn't already), and if she is afraid to talk to her mom, encourage her to talk to your own mom. A parent will have more experience with this type of problem and will have ideas about getting the appropriate help for her. Your friend will need to talk to a health care professional to make sure she is healthy and that she wasn't physically hurt. If your friend is afraid to see a doctor or nurse, you may offer to go with her. Reassure your friend that secrecy breeds shame. What happened to her is not her fault, but it is her responsibility to make sure she is okay and that the same thing doesn't happen to another innocent person.

> TABLE TALK:
>
> **Table Talk Conversation about Concern over Friends.**
> *For this example of what you might say when concerned about your friend, you could try this. Let's pretend you are Sue and your friend is Leila.*
>
> *Sue: Leila, I am worried about you.*
>
> *Leila: Don't worry, I'm fine.*
>
> *Sue: You don't act the same, ever since he forced you to have sex. You look sad, and you are always preoccupied. You don't laugh anymore. (Say anything you have noticed that appears different from her "old behavior.")*
>
> *Leila: I am just tired. I am stressed out with school. Really, don't worry.*
>
> *Sue: Leila, you cannot handle this on your own. You need to go get checked to make sure you aren't suffering from him hurting you. You need to be tested Leila. How about if we talk to my mom?*
>
> *Leila: No, she will tell my mom and my mom will be so angry. She will not understand and she will think I did it or caused it.*

Sue: Leila, I will be with you. Let's start with my mom and she will know what is best to do. We have to do it now. You could have gotten a disease or an infection. The more you wait the worse it will become.

Leila: I'm scared. I don't want to deal with this. I think I will be okay.

Sue: Let's just start by talking to my mom. We will take it one day at a time from there and see what happens. I will stay with you... and I promise I will go through this with you.

The most important thing for Sue to do is to reassure her friend that she will not leave her side. She will not judge her or think less of her no matter what. If Leila knows she has a good friend by her side, that will help her be stronger. If Sue can get her mom to help with Leila and Leila's mom, that will be the best support for both girls.

Q: What are steps I can do to stay safe on dates or when out with a group of friends?

A: The safest way to stay safe with a group is to stay with the group. Tell your parents whom you will be with and where you will be. Have phone numbers of all your friends (and their parent's name) as a reference list for your parents to keep. Don't ever leave your friends when you go out with them. Don't ever let one of your friends leave the group without telling them you will call either their parent or your own parent (friends never let friends leave alone).

When you go out with your friends make sure it is clear *up front* that you will all leave as a group together. This past summer in Houston this very issue led to the death of a young girl. She had gone out with a group of her friends. Two boys came whom the girl knew, but none of her friends knew the two guys well or at all. The girl left with the two boys (her friends let her go because they had not set up a *pact* or agreement prior to going out). The girl ended up never coming home. Her body was found two days later and the boys who had killed her were arrested soon thereafter. When they asked the boys what had provoked them to do such a heinous act one of them casually replied he wanted to know what it felt like to kill someone. Can you imagine what kind of a person would say this, or do this? We may never fully comprehend why.

The bottom line is a young girl is dead who could still have been alive if she hadn't left without her friends, or if her friends had called her mother. Be a good friend; if you come with a friend (or friends), go home with your friend (or friends).

Q: My friend is in a relationship with a boy she wants to break up with, but every time she talks to him about breaking up he tells her if she does he will kill himself. How should she break up with him?

A: Wow. Talk about a low self-esteem. This guy needs help! Your friend is involved with someone who is so emotionally fragile that he feels he cannot exist with out her. She should not flatter herself. This guy needs someone, and my guess is that if it isn't your friend it will be someone else. He is using her.

Many times, when boys or girls say this they are crying for help. Your friend may believe it is because she is irreplaceable to him. This is usually not the case. Your friend should tell her mom exactly what she told you. She should definitely break up the relationship as this is a sign of an unhealthy relationship. When she breaks up with him she should tell her mom and also the boy's mother. That way, if he is serious his mom will be aware of what is going on and can take steps to help him deal with his grief.

It is *never* a good sign to be in a relationship where one of the individuals feels like they cannot survive without the other. This could also be a way for your friend's boyfriend to control her. Think about it: should anyone who cares about you be this desperate to control you? Your friend's relationship is not healthy; neither person is able to grow and develop normally. It would be a good idea for him to have counseling, and your friend might also benefit to help her understand why she remained in such an unhealthy relationship. The counselor could also give her steps or warning signs to prevent this happening in the future.

Q: My friend is head over heels in love with a boy. He shows little interest in her, but she changes or reframes conversations he may have with her to make it look like he is infatuated with her. How can I help my friend?

A: Your friend is going through what we all go through at least once and maybe several times. It is a version of obsession and it is directed at a boy she really likes. Your friend wants to believe that she is important to this boy because she really likes him. He may or may not like her, but most likely he does not feel the same way she does. The best thing you can do is to always be honest with her about what you see. Continually express her assets and validate how special she is to you. She may need to feel better about herself and feel like she is attractive. She will eventually let go if nothing comes of it, but right now she needs to hear that no matter how he feels, you think she is great, and that she is a wonderful friend. It is always good to tell a friend who did not get "chosen" by the guy she really liked that it was his oversight. Your friend is great!

MOM QUESTIONS

Now let's entertain some questions from mothers about *sexuality and relationships*. Tough questions, tough issues; definitely worthwhile table talk conversations.

Q: You mentioned sacro sex. What is? How can I teach my daughter about it?

A: I am so glad you asked that question. *Sacro sex* is the concept that sexuality is a sacred union—a coming together of intense intimacy. It is built, not simply "engaged in." It starts out with a friendship and grows into a relationship that can endure hardships and setbacks. *Sacro sex* perseveres because it is not engaged in hastily; it takes time to build. To teach your daughter about *sacro sex* would mean you would teach her the importance of friendships. It would mean that you would model what it means to be a good friend. It means you would refrain from exposing her to gossip or betrayal of friendship. *Sacro sex* is a result of a long term friendship and relationship with someone. *Sacro sex* means valuing the other person as much as you value yourself so you don't manipulate that person or take advantage of his or her feelings. Precisely because *sacro sex* is "sacro", it cannot be engaged in until both people have attained an age of emotional maturity, which usually develops *after* physical maturity occurs. Our experience is that this emotional maturity does not come before age eighteen. *Sacro sex* is setting a high standard for yourself and the person you love. It means you value the relationship and therefore have considered the consequences of engaging in any behavior that could jeopardize the relationship.

Q: My daughter wants to go to a party with friends I don't know well. Is there anything I can do to help ensure her safety?

A: The answer to this question depends very much on your child. Is your child trustworthy? Do you have good communication between the two of you? If your child is under the age of sixteen I would let her go to the party, but I would structure a pick up time when I would come to pick her up. I would make sure that the party was at someone's house whose parents were going to be home. I would have the parents' phone number and call them in advance. If your child can drive, I would still set a curfew time beforehand when I expected her home.

I would make sure the party was supervised by adults, and I would have a physical address of where the party was and a contact (i.e., parent) phone number. I would have a list of three of the children who would be there with phone numbers (if she doesn't have their phone numbers then she doesn't know them well enough to go to the party). Again, my biggest concern is always my daughter's safety. This is your chance to be a *mom*. Not a buddy or someone who is cool. Rather, someone who has experience and wisdom and strength to set strong boundaries so your daughter will be able to feel supported by your structure.

Q: Are there steps I can take to help my daughter not have sex before the age of eighteen?

A: The best steps to prevent sex before the age of eighteen involve good communication between you and your daughter. Being a mom means wanting what is best for your child. That includes building their self-esteem so they see all of their gifts clearly. It means respecting their boundaries, their friendships, and listening to them. Many times girls have sex to keep a boyfriend around. They feel like the boyfriend gives them attention and they crave this because they never got it from home.

Talk to your daughter about your own views. She respects you and wants to know. If you can be a strong and confident woman she will feel like it is possible for her to be also. If girls feel like there are no limits to learning and contributing to the greater good of the community, they will not focus as much on the status of having a boyfriend. Support your daughter in her interests. Encourage her to become involved in her community, sports, giving back. The girls who are at risk for having sex before the age of eighteen are girls who grow up looking for someone else (a boy) to make them feel loved and important. Teach your daughter to develop her own interests and passions rather than looking for someone else to fill this need for her.

Q: I just found out my sixteen year old is having sex with a boy who is twenty-one. Is this legal and what should I do?

A: The last part of your question I will answer first. *No, it is almost never legal* and you should get legal advice to deal with this question. I would sit down with my daughter and talk to her about your concerns in regard to this situation.

Secondly, what is she getting from this relationship? Is she getting enough attention from her dad? It sounds like this may be an area of concern. At any rate, I would not tolerate it. I would try to start spending more time with my daughter. I would listen to her more, find ways she could express her feelings (this may involve counseling). This type of situation is usually a symptom of problems in a family. Most likely it has to do with your daughter feeling alone and unprotected.

Family counseling may be beneficial as it sounds like boundaries could be an issue in your family. Is it possible that your daughter doesn't feel loved or secure, or that she doesn't feel strong in who she is? This twenty-one year old man obviously has intimacy issues, and if it were my daughter, I would go to the authorities.

Q: What do I do if I don't like the boy my daughter is head over heels for?

A: It is easier to tell you what not to do. Do not make a rule that states she cannot see him. If your daughter feels like you don't like him she will most likely cling to him tighter to protect him. It is a wise tactic to try and embrace the boy more. Invite him to dinner with his parents. This helps on two levels. The first is you get to see him with his family and determine if his family is respectful. You can also see family dynamics and whether there are tensions in the family. Secondly, you will make your daughter less defensive. She will not have to work so hard to protect him. She will be able to compare him and his family to her own. Usually this helps to give her a clearer idea of whether she really likes him. You may find you have misjudged him, and maybe you will see characteristics in him that you actually respect.

If you are concerned (for any reason) about the way he treats your daughter, the best time to bring that sort of discussion up is when the two of you are alone. Have a quiet and comfortable environment and start out by asking her how she feels about him. Really listen to her, and when she discloses any areas of concern this would be a good time to interject your concerns. If she feels like you are not going to criticize her or her boyfriend she will be more likely to tell you things she is not happy with. I have a lot of faith in young women. They are so much more intuitive and wiser then I ever remember being. If you think your daughter is, given a quiet place to talk with a parent whom she feels is really on her side, she will tell you more than you ever imagined. If your daughter is aware that you love her and only want what is best for her, she will usually be very patient with your anxieties. Every mother wants to protect her daughter from heartbreak or worse. The problem is, sometimes the heartbreak is inevitable and is the only way your daughter can learn the really hard lessons from a relationship.

Q: But what if I like the boy, maybe even more than my daughter does? Shouldn't I try to keep him around?

A: I love your question because it happened to me with my own daughter. It is difficult because we know our daughters so well, and we can identify when someone really appreciates them and treats them with respect. The problem is that we don't see them all the time. Sometimes (most of the time in my own case) my daughter will have better insight into who treats her well and who doesn't. I think the best solution is to try and treat all of your daughter's friends with respect. She is watching you, and you are mentoring respect for her. If there is a boyfriend you are concerned about, you should definitely speak to your daughter about him, but if there is someone she is somewhat "cool about" and you think he hung the moon, respect your daughter's way of dealing with him. She probably sees things about him that you do not.

Q: Sometimes I am worried about possible danger with the Internet or text messaging. How can I stress the importance of safety when my daughter sees this as a way of life?

A: This is an important question and one with which most of us struggle. My answer goes back to the importance of having open communication between you and your daughter. Most of the dangerous things that happen related to the Internet and instant messaging happen to girls who feel alone or isolated. If you are there for your daughter and constantly sit with her and talk about these issues, it should pose much less of a risk. I do limit the computer and cell phone in the evening. No computer (except for homework) after 10:00 p.m. No cell phones past 10:30 p.m. This took work on my part because I had to be there to enforce the rule. That was a small price to pay for being able to sleep at night.

Q: My daughter keeps trying to "fit in" with the popular kids. These children are not nice to her nor do they respect me or our family rules. What should I do?

A: This is a difficult dilemma. One of the problems is that when your daughter is older than twelve, you have little influence over who she wants to be friends with. Usually if you try to discourage her, she will be upset and angry at you and will want to befriend these people even more. I would advise that you keep the lines of communication open so that your daughter can continue to talk about what she is experiencing and she can tell you when these friends hurt her or cause her emotional pain.

I also usually encourage moms to join forces with other moms. Maybe someone else in the group is having the same feelings you are. When your daughter sees you are making an effort to join the moms of friends she respects, she may be able to feel more honest and open about what is going on. Maybe your daughter feels less worthy or has feelings of insecurity that she believes will go away if she is with the popular kids. We all know that this will not happen; in fact, she may find that she feels worse about herself because the popular kids are often not as thoughtful or respectful of others. The more you are able to communicate with your daughter all of the wonderful things you see in her, the more she will become confident in herself and the more she will resist people who do not have her own or others' best interest at heart.

Q: My daughter is very isolated. She has no "real friends" in whom she feels she can confide, nor does she like to participate in activities on the weekends. How can I help her branch our more and socialize?

A: I hate to hear this. It could signify an underlying depression or grief process. The first thing I would suggest is making an appointment with a counselor and going together with your daughter. If you are new in town or don't know of a good counselor, I would suggest you talk with a teacher, school counselor or your family doctor.

If you have just moved, this could be the process of starting a new school in a new area. If not, it may be that your daughter is changing or something has precipitated this isolation. It is important that you talk to her. It may be helpful to discuss a time when you felt like this. Share with her what you did. Listen to suggestions or ideas she has. Feeling blue is a normal part of being an adolescent girl, but continuing to feel blue longer then two weeks or to become isolated from friends and social interaction is not normal. You must explore her feelings in order to help her.

Life is not measured by the number of breaths we take, but by the moments that take our breath away.

-George Carlin

CHAPTER 5

"Mom, I Need to Tell You Something."

BIRTH CONTROL

One of the major reasons for writing this book is the amount of unintended pregnancy that we witness on many occasions. We have witnessed adoption, abortion, girls becoming single parents, and young couples getting married. We have seen every outcome and, although people go on with their lives, each decision is difficult.

Many young girls become pregnant because they think they can't, so they don't use birth control. Others never think about the consequences. But most of the time it happens to the girl who is wanting to use only abstinence as her method of birth control. The thought of abstinence is a wonderful one; we support it. Yet the fact is that many people who say they are committed to abstinence truly want to be, but often are not. Since most abstinence programs do not discuss birth control, many girls are completely unprepared for or not capable of coming to terms with the need for birth control when they choose *not* to abstain.

Recent studies have indicated that 88% of people have premarital sex. If you are a virgin now, it is likely that before you get married you will probably have intercourse. Unintended pregnancy is difficult no matter what your age. However, for an unmarried teen it can be much more difficult. No matter what the outcome, life is never the same. The full impact may not be realized for years to come.

My first experience with unintended pregnancy was in college. I had a close friend who had a steady boyfriend, and in her heart she did not want to be sexually active. But over time the relationship became sexual. Many of her friends could see that she was heading down that path just by things she would tell us. When the idea of birth control would come up her response was that she would not "get on the pill" because she knew if she did that she would probably give in and have intercourse. She did not want to do that. She believed that "sex" was right only if you were married.

Everyone around her knew that there were heavy make-out sessions, since she and her boyfriend would disappear for hours behind locked doors. We did not believe they were "just studying." Again, every time we brought up the idea of birth control she dismissed it. We suggested that if she were trying to abstain, then maybe she shouldn't put herself in the position where she could reach a point of no return.

Finally, one day she confided in me that she thought she was late for her period. She had concerns that she might be pregnant. We ran to the local pharmacy, performed a home pregnancy test and — to no one's surprise — it was positive. She was devastated, to say the least, and was worried about telling her boyfriend. Although they had been dating for a number of months, he made it clear he was not ready for a long term commitment. Finally she told him. Although he promised to help, the only feasible option he felt they had was for her to terminate the pregnancy.

Devastation hardly describes the reaction my friend had to this idea. First of all, she was someone who had an extremely difficult time with the idea of premarital sex for religious reasons; abortion clearly did not seem like something that she could do. Her boyfriend told her that he was definitely not ready for marriage and fatherhood was simply out of the question. He offered to take her for the termination — even pay for it. I am not certain if the idea of adoption was ever even discussed. He took her to another state for the procedure, since in 1980 that was where the closest abortions were being performed.

She described going to the clinic and having to walk though protest lines in order to get through the door and how hard that was as she herself had problems with the idea of having an abortion. Her boyfriend stayed with her until it was time to go back for the procedure. She pleaded with him to no avail to think of another way. She went through with the procedure, was given a pack of birth control pills to start, and went back to her life. After the termination she continued to see him and decided again that she would go back to abstinence as her method of birth control, choosing not to start on the pill. They soon became sexually active again, and with much persuasion from many friends, she finally got on the pill.

Years later, every time I spoke with her, the termination would still come up. I'm not sure that she has ever truly come to terms with her decision. Looking back as a health care professional it became clear to me how preventable this situation was. Believing that abstinence was the best path became a dangerous choice when she was unable to match that with her emotions. I am all for abstinence; however, I am also for honesty with yourself. If you are unable to abstain, use protection because the consequences are much worse should you become pregnant.

Let's take a few minutes to talk about birth control, as a background to our question/answer discussion. There are many different types of birth control — both hormonal and non hormonal. *Non hormonal* includes:

1. **Abstinence**—complete avoidance of sexual intercourse, which is the most efficacious way to prevent pregnancy, but it is not effective if you don't abstain.

2. **Natural Family Planning**—a method of birth control often instituted by couples who don't want to use a hormonal or barrier method of birth control. It is based on not having intercourse at the point in a woman's cycle that she is most able to get pregnant. There are many ways to utilize natural family planning. Some of the methods to assist in determining fertile times of the month are the calendar method, cervical mucus, and temperature charts. Natural family planning requires a great deal of education and great knowledge of your menstrual cycles, as well as willpower to resist sexual intercourse.

3. **Withdrawal**—withdrawing the penis prior to ejaculation. One of the least effective methods of birth control, more than 25% of women will get pregnant by using withdrawal as their primary method. To be effective, withdrawal requires great control by the man since there can be a large number of sperm in the pre-ejaculation fluid.

4. **Male condoms**—a thin latex sheath that covers the penis during sexual intercourse. If used consistently, they are quite effective against pregnancy and sexually transmitted infections. A specific advantage is that you can buy them without a prescription. The biggest problem is that they often are not used properly or they are used inconsistently. Condoms can be made from "natural" substances other than latex, but these can be less effective to prevent STDs.

5. **Female condoms**—a polyurethane barrier that is inserted into the woman's vagina. They are less effective than the male condom in preventing pregnancy and sexually transmitted infections. They can be cumbersome to insert, especially for young girls who are uncomfortable with touching their genital area. They are expensive, but can be bought over the counter.

6. **Spermicide**—that comes in various forms such suppositories, foams, and creams that work by immobilizing sperm. The typical failure rate is nearly 30%, but used in conjunction with condoms it increases the effectiveness of the birth control method as well as preventing

STDs. They can be bought over the counter. A major problem is that spermicides can be very irritating to the vagina.

7. Sponge—a barrier method made of a solid polyurethane sponge that is saturated with spermicide. Typical pregnancy rates for women who have never been pregnant and who use a sponge are approximately 15%. The rates in women who have been pregnant before are approximately double. The sponge is inserted deep into the vagina prior to intercourse and can stay in the vagina for a period of time and still be effective. Sponges can be bought without a prescription.

8. Diaphragm—is a firm rimmed shallow cup that is inserted into the vagina over the cervix. It is used in conjunction with spermicidal agents. The diaphragm is bought only with a prescription and requires a health care provider to fit the patient with the proper size. It is generally not a popular method in the teen population due to the importance of good placement for it to work. The typical effectiveness rate in women who have never been pregnant is approximately 85%.

Hormonal methods do not protect against STDs but can be effective to prevent pregnancy. They include:

1. Combination oral contraceptive pills—the most commonly prescribed method of birth control in teen girls. These pills contain both estrogen and progesterone. All of the pills contain the same estrogen, called ethenyl estradiol, but at different doses. There are several different types of progesterones that also can be at different doses.

Oral contraceptives come in two types: *monophasic pills*, where the dose is the same everyday, and *triphasic pills*, where the dose varies each day to try to be more like your natural cycle.

Traditional pill packs contain three weeks of active pills and one week of placebo or sugar pills. The pill works by giving the woman's body the types of hormones that the ovaries would normally make, thus taking away the need for the pituitary to stimulate the ovaries. Take away that stimulation and the ovaries will not ovulate. The pill also thickens the mucus covering the cervix, which makes it more difficult for sperm to enter the uterus and thins out the lining of the uterus which can prevent implantation.

The placebo allows your hormone levels to drop just like in a normal cycle, which is when you generally will start your period. During the last several years, there have been several new formulations. For example, some of the new pills have 24 days of active pills and four days of sugar pills. This arrangement is thought to suppress more completely ovarian function. Studies have shown that when you take seven days of sugar pills, ovarian function returns on day five. These pills also produce cycles that tend to be shorter and lighter.

There are also pills that have 12 weeks of active pills and one week of placebos, giving you cycles every three months. Recently, a new pill has come out with no sugar pills. The problem with these two types of pills is that there can be some irregular bleeding, which can be very frustrating.

Perfect use of the pill offers greater than 99% effectiveness. The biggest problem with teens and the pills is remembering to take them. If you don't take them properly, the effectiveness rates can fall considerably.

There are a few important risks with the pill; therefore, it requires an accurate personal and family history prior to starting the pill. If you have a personal history of a blood clot or a strong family history of blood clots, you should not take the pill. Smoking also increases risks associated with the pill — another great reason not to start smoking at all! In rare cases, estrogen can raise blood pressure.

2. **Patch**—worn on the skin and changed weekly. It can be great for girls who don't take the pill regularly. A new patch is put on once a week for three weeks, and on the fourth week you do not use the patch. This is when you will have your period. The problem with the patch is that there is some question about how smoothly the delivery system of the hormones works. Therefore, I rarely prescribe it unless I have no other option and I feel that getting pregnant is likely to happen if the woman doesn't use the patch.

3. **Vaginal ring**—a round flexible ring that can easily be inserted into the vagina like a tampon. It also contains estrogen and progesterone. Exact placement isn't important like it is with the diaphragm. The ring stays in place for three weeks and is taken out for one week, which is

when you will have your period. It contains the lowest dose of estrogen of any combined hormonal contraception. Two great features of the ring are: You don't have to remember it daily and hormone levels stay very even. Many teens who are comfortable enough with their body to insert the ring are very satisfied with it.

4. Progestin-only pills—contraceptive pills that contain only progesterone. They work by thickening the cervical mucus and preventing sperm from entering the uterine cavity. The effectiveness depends on taking the pill regularly to keep the cervical mucus thickened. Often, people who use this method will not have regular cycles.

5. Depo Provera—a birth control method that is given through an injection every 12 weeks. It is a type of synthetic progesterone. It is a very effective method of birth control that works by suppressing ovulation, thickening the cervical mucus and thinning the lining of the uterus. The advantage of this method is that it only has to be thought about every three months but it can have many side effects that girls do not like. Weight gain and PMS are the most commonly reported side effects. Furthermore, it offers no protection against STDs. Long term use can cause a decrease in bone formation, so using it longer than three years is discouraged. Adequate calcium is extremely important in this age group.

All of these methods are equally effective against pregnancy but are not effective in the prevention of STDs. The combination of a hormonal method with a condom is the best method to prevent both pregnancy and sexually transmitted infections.

There are some other methods as well:

Inter-uterine devices are inserted into the uterine cavity. Some contain hormones, and some do not. Both types work by thickening the cervical mucus, thereby preventing sperm from getting into the uterine cavity. They *do not* work by causing abortions. Generally, they are used in women who are in monogamous relationships and who have given birth.

Another method is an implantable rod (about the size of a match stick) that is inserted under the skin on the upper arm, usually with local anesthesia. It stays in place for three years and is greater than 99.9% effective in preventing pregnancy. It works similarly to Depo Provera, since it contains another synthetic progesterone. The implantable rod is very new so there is not a lot of information about long-term use. Most teens do not want to use methods that require insertion. However, it can be used in people who can not use estrogen-containing methods due to side effects. It does not offer protection against STDs.

There is a type of *emergency contraception* (EC) that can be given within 120 hours of sexual intercourse. EC works when another method was not used or a problem with that method was encountered. For example, if the condom breaks or withdrawal did not occur in enough time, EC can be used. The earlier you use EC, the more effective it will be. It can reduce pregnancy rates by 75-89%. EC works by stopping ovulation or fertilization but it generally will not stop a pregnancy that has already occurred.

The most common type of EC is made up of a combination of hormones at high doses. Plan B, a brand of EC, has been approved by the FDA to be available without a prescription for women over the age of 18. Girls under the age of 18 will still need a prescription. It is kept behind the pharmacy counter and not all pharmacies carry it. This method has been controversial with some conservative groups since it is thought to cause abortions. In rare cases, a copper IUD will be placed for emergency contraception.

So let's move to some table-talk conversations about birth control. How about some Q&A on birth control? Daughters, why don't we address your questions first?

DAUGHTER QUESTIONS

Q: Are there days during your cycle that you are most likely to get pregnant?

A: Depending on the length of your cycle, ovulation generally occurs about 14 days before starting your period. For example, if you have 28-day cycles, you are probably ovulating on day 14. A few things to keep in mind are that if your cycles vary in length, ovulation won't always be on day 14. Also, remember that sperm can live for up to

72 hours, so if you have unprotected intercourse on day 12 and you ovulate on day 14 you can get pregnant from the sperm that have been hanging around for two days.

Q: Why is withdrawal not an effective method of birth control?

A: Withdrawal method of birth control can be very risky since there can be a large number of sperm in the pre-ejaculation fluid that can be released without knowledge. Especially in young men who don't have good control of ejaculation, it can be quite risky to use this as a primary method of birth control

Q: Can you really get pregnant the first time you have unprotected sex?

A: YES, YES and YES! Often, girls get pregnant the first time they have intercourse due to the hormonal changes that occur around ovulation, leading them to say "yes" to intercourse in the heat of the moment. Remember *Welcome to Menstruation 101*: your body is waiting and wanting sperm around ovulation. All you need to get pregnant is an egg and sperm, so if the timing is right, it doesn't matter if it is your first time or your hundredth time.

Q: Does the birth control pill cause infertility?

A: No, the pill does not cause infertility, and in some cases may help prevent problems with fertility by minimizing endometriosis and ovarian cysts. No one will know your exact fertility until you try to get pregnant (or try *not* to get pregnant), but the pill does not make you infertile. When you stop the pill, it may take a few months for the ovaries to wake up and ovulate. A one-to-three month "wake-up" span is not unusual. Remember that some women may take pills to treat an underlying condition that itself can cause infertility, like irregular periods or endometriosis.

Q: What is the average amount of weight gain from birth control pills?

A: This is the number one question asked by teens when placed on hormonal birth control. Many studies looking at weight gain on the pill have been done over the years. On the older, higher dose pills there were reports of weight gain averaging five pounds. Studies done with newer, lower dose pills show less than a two-pound weight gain in total; the majority of people actually gained no weight and some even lost a few pounds. In general, the low dose pills are considered weight neutral.

In my practice, I see patients back after three months on the pill to check their weight and blood pressure. I rarely see a significant change in either, but if I do, I begin to explore if their eating habits have changed. Every once in a while a patient will report that she is eating more, but it is very rare. If there is a change in her appetite I will switch to a different pill to see if there is a difference.

Q: Can the birth control pill cause my moodiness to get worse?

A: The birth control pill can make your moods get much worse or much better. There are studies that looked at the effect of the birth control pill on PMS. Since the pill can even out your hormones, it can improve PMS and moods significantly. In combination birth control pills, the same type of estrogen is used but in varying amounts. What is most different among pills is the type of progestin they contain. There are basically three types of progestin, and they can affect your mood a great deal.

Therefore, if you are feeling increased moodiness, anxiety, or tearfulness after you begin your oral contraceptives, you need to notify your medical office. The best way to try to improve your mood with the pill is to change the type of progestin. Most of the time, you can find a pill that does not make your mood worse and one that can help get rid of PMS. So if taking the pill leaves you feeling like your "evil twin" has taken over your body, talk with your health care provider about switching to a different kind of pill.

Q: At what age is it safe for girls to start birth control pills?

A: There is not a recommended age for you to start the pill. Each person uses the pill for different reasons. Girls who are as young as 12, with extremely heavy or irregular cycles, have been placed on the pill to control their periods with great success. Dermatologists sometimes request a trial of birth control prior to Accutane® use and some dermatologists will require birth control before using the drug because of the risk of birth defects induced by Accutane®. Age generally will not be the reason that someone won't be placed on the pill.

Q: How can you skip periods with the pill, and is it safe to do so?

A: One of the people who helped create the birth control pill said that the biggest mistake made in the birth control pack was not eliminating the monthly period. The sugar pill week was put in to allow your period to start, and it was put in monthly to mimic a monthly period. You do not have to have a monthly period, and it is safe to skip periods by starting a new pack when you come to the sugar pills. There are pills that go 12 weeks without a sugar pill week. The problem that can occur is that you can start having irregular periods if you go too long without a period.

Many young girls who have very heavy cycles cannot go many weeks without having breakthrough bleeding. Generally, the longer you can go without irregular bleeding on extended pills, the longer you will be able to go without a period. You don't build up excess lining because the uterine lining is made inactive by birth control pills. Some periods on extended pills can be a bit heavy, but in general they are not bad. The newer pills have only four days of sugar pills, so periods become very light and, hopefully, uneventful.

Q: What part of the cycle is the best time to start taking birth control pills, and when are they effective?

A: The best day to start your pills is the first day of your cycle, which is defined as the first day of menstrual bleeding. Not only will this lighten up your period, but you will also have immediate birth control. The other time to start your pill is the Sunday after the first day of your period. For example, if you start your cycle on Thursday, you will start the pill three days later. But, if you start the pill at least 24 hours after the beginning of your period, you need to use a back up method of birth control for one week.

Q: What is the proper way to take birth control pills?

A: After starting a combination birth control pill, it is important to take it regularly. It doesn't matter what time of day you take your pill, but you need to be somewhat consistent. For example, if you take it every morning before school, generally around 8:00 am, but you sleep in a little later on the weekend, then take it as soon as you wake up. Same thing if you take it at night. Forgetting doses or taking one pill in the morning today and another tomorrow night will only cause you problems with bleeding, PMS, and even the possibility that it won't be effective. Everyone at some point will forget a pill; however, you need to try to be as regular as possible in taking them. Some people keep it with their toothbrush, and every time they brush they take the pill. Make it a routine.

Q: What is the morning-after pill?

A: The morning after pill is another term for Emergency Contraception used in preventing pregnancy when you didn't use birth control. For girls over 18, it can be bought at many pharmacies without a prescription. It is also used to prevent pregnancy after rape has occurred.

Q: Are girls who take birth control more likely to have sex earlier?

A: This question is so frequently asked—it is wonderful you asked. There is no evidence that girls who take birth control are more likely to have sex. In fact, it is usually just the opposite. Girls who take birth control pills understand that it has other health benefits besides preventing pregnancy. They may take it for help to control heavy or uncomfortable periods, to relieve acne, or so periods don't interfere with life's activities such as athletic competitions.

Many times, girls who are sexually active are ashamed to admit they are having sex. They feel like they have to hide it and, therefore, they do not use birth control. They are afraid of talking to their moms about their sexual activities, so they never mention that they may need protection. They may take more risks in general with other areas of their life as well. In my counseling practice, it is the girls who aren't educated in regard to birth control and aren't using birth control who are more likely to be sexually active.

Q: *What are reasons I should consider taking the birth control pill?*

A: There are a number of reasons girls start birth control. Many times, it is related to menstrual problems such as irregular, painful, or heavy cycles. There are medical problems that can be improved with birth control pills, such acne, PMS, ovarian cysts or endometriosis, just to name a few. Of course, if you are considering becoming sexually active, the pill is a contraceptive option. But, remember, it doesn't protect against STDs.

Lucy, a 16-year old girl, came into my office with her mother, Janie. Lucy's dermatologist had recommended that Lucy begin taking birth control pills before she started a new acne medicine that could, if she became pregnant, cause birth defects in her child.

Lucy, her mother and I sat in the exam room and discussed how Lucy should start taking the birth control pills. While we talked, I noted that Janie frequently answered my questions even before Lucy could start to speak. Her mother even commented that she could not understand why Lucy needed to be on birth control pills just to take the acne medication because Lucy had never been sexually active. I sensed that Lucy was uncomfortable with this discussion.

I realized that it would be a good idea to talk to Lucy without her mother in the room. Once Lucy and I were alone, I asked her if there was anything that she wanted to add to her health history. She fidgeted, did not look at me directly, and then nodded her head yes. When I asked her if she had been sexually active, she responded "well, sort of." Eventually she told me that she had sexual intercourse a "couple of times" with the 18-year-old boy whom she had been dating for six months, and that they had not used any form of protection from either pregnancy or sexually transmitted infections. Lucy added that her mother would "kill her" if she found out that she had been having sex with her boyfriend.

I questioned whether she ever spoke about sex with her mother, and she told me that neither of them ever brought up the subject. Lucy said that she was certain that her mother expected her to remain a virgin until she got married.

We talked about the possible consequences of unprotected sexual activity. I encouraged her to practice safe sex, or at least to get tested for sexually transmitted diseases (STDs)— along with her partner. I explained to Lucy that she would need to have a gynecologic exam soon. Although I recommended that she open up and tell her mother about her sexual activity, I assured her that our discussion was confidential, and I promised that I would not say anything to her mother about it. I prescribed a low dose birth control pill with instructions on how to take it. As I handed her my card with the date of her next appointment, I encouraged her to call me at any time if she wanted to talk. I reminded her that, despite the conflict, her mother remained an important resource for her as well.

Q: What if the condom breaks during sexual intercourse?

A: If you used no other method of birth control, then you should call your health care professional for emergency contraception. If you are over 18, you can get EC at a pharmacy without a prescription. If you used another method of birth control along with the condom, and your concern is STDs, then get tested for STDs.

Q: What age do I have to be to buy a condom?

A: There is no age restriction to purchase condoms. In most pharmacies they are kept out in the open where they are easy to get. At many college campuses they are available for free in the student health center.

Q: How do I ask my mom about birth control? How should I tell her I want to be on the pill?

A: This is a good question. You may need to preface your question with why you want to go on the pill. Do you want to start the pill to help improve the way you feel prior to your periods? Do you want to go on the pill to help control an acne break-out? Your mom may be fearful of your intentions. She may think you want to have sex or she may feel like you are growing up too fast. All of these things will make her react, and she may not listen well when you first bring it up. Therefore, I suggest you ask her when you can talk to her about something important so she will set time aside and be there for you completely. If you ask her spontaneously while she is doing something else, she may overreact. This is an opportunity for you and your mom to get closer. Below is a suggestion of how you may bring it up.

TABLE TALK

Table Talk Conversation on Bringing up the Subject of Birth Control.

You: Mom, can I have some time to talk with you about something that has been on my mind?

Mom: What is it, what's the matter?

You: It's nothing bad mom, relax. I just need your advice, and I want your guidance with something I am thinking about.

Mom: Oh, okay, can we do it tomorrow as soon as I get home from work?

You: That will be great. Where should we meet?

Mom: How about if we meet each other at the kitchen table at 5:30 p.m.?

You: Perfect.

(Congratulations daughter, you have set the table. Mom will be ready to listen, and you can explain what you need from her).

Q: How likely am I to get a blood clot from being on the pill?

A: Very unlikely. Girls who take birth control pills have a 15-20/100,000 chance of developing a blood clot. Even women who don't take the pill have a 5/100,000 chance of developing a blood clot. Keep in mind that pregnancy raises the risk of blood clot even higher than being on the pill. It is important to tell the person prescribing the pill if you have a personal or strong family history of blood clots. If there is a strong family history, I often send a patient to a hematologist to have the risk evaluated. Smoking also increases your risk of blood clots.

Q: How do birth control pills differ and how do I know if I am on the right pill?

A: Combination birth control pills all have the same type of estrogen hormone, ethinyl estradiol, but in varying amounts generally ranging from 20mcg-35mcg. There are higher dose pills, but these are not typically prescribed to new pill users. There are different types of progestins (the progesterone part of the pill). Generally, if a pill gives you a side effect such as PMS, try a pill with a different progestin.

Most pill packs prescribed today have 28 pills, but there are 21- and 93-pill packs. Placebo or sugar pills range from 4-7 days in each pack. For a new user, I usually pick a 20mcg monophasic 28-day pill. The best way to know if you are on the right pill is to let your symptoms be your guide. If you feel well, have regular cycles after the first few months, haven't developed or worsened PMS, have no weight gain, normal blood pressure, and menstrual symptoms are improved, then you are probably on the right pill. I have new users come back in three months to check their blood pressure and weight, and to discuss any noted side effects, symptoms or problems. Jointly we determine if the pill is the correct one. If it isn't the right one, we will make a change at that time. Also, remember, you do not need to have a pelvic exam.

Q: I am afraid to tell my parents I may be pregnant. They are going to "kill me!"

A: First things first: It's incredibly unlikely that parents would kill their daughter because they found out she was pregnant. They may become very upset, but they most likely will not kill you. If you are really worried about your physical safety, I suggest asking the school nurse, a teacher, a guidance counselor, or a coach to accompany you when you tell them. Remember, your parents may be frustrated and upset, or even angry at themselves (which will probably get projected onto you). When you first tell them, they will be shocked and may be immediately reactive. Give them time. Remember, you have probably suspected it for a while, but they will need some time to think and consider appropriate options.

Q: How do I decide if I should terminate a pregnancy?

A: First of all, preventing pregnancy is the best way not to have to make this decision. But, assuming you have become pregnant, this is a very personal question that only you can answer. We have watched girls make every decision from abortion, to adoption, to having and raising the child. It is the woman's choice, since she will have to ultimately live with whatever choice is made.

The decision to terminate or not to terminate will be with you forever. It is important, if you are facing this decision, to talk to a trusted adult. If you feel that you are not ready to tell your parents, talk to a teacher, counselor or health care professional. As a health care provider, I have been in the situation where I have helped a young girl tell her parents. It is important to understand all of your options and to explore your true feelings. Again, prevention is the key.

TABLE TALK

Table Talk Conversation on Possible Pregnancy. Here is a suggestion of how you may want to bring this up with your mom. If you have a pretty good relationship with her, you may want to talk to her alone first and then with your dad. Before you start, make sure you have allowed yourself time. You don't want to be stressed or "moody" before the talk, as you will need to be able to think of what you want to say. Just like I said earlier, if you are worried about your safety, then go to another adult woman before your mom. She may want to accompany you when you tell your mom. Let's pretend your name is Jenny, so below would be the conversation.

Jenny: Mom, I have something to tell you and I am afraid to say it.

Mom: What is it? Tell me, you don't have to be afraid.

Jenny: Mom, I am afraid because I love you so much, and I am afraid you are going to be angry or so disappointed with me. I cannot take that, and I hate to hurt your feelings.

Mom: What is it? Let's sit down. (Mom may put her arm around you; if she doesn't, take HER hand.)

Jenny: I think I might be pregnant and I am really scared.

Mom: Oh, My God! (Give mom time here... remember she has heard it for the first time, and she will be hurt, scared, angry, guilty).

Jenny: I am sorry, Mom. I didn't think it would happen.

Mom: How late are you?

Jenny: I am six weeks past my last period.

Mom: How did this happen? How could you... after all I told you?

Jenny: (Breathe deep ... Be calm. Give mom time. She is worried for you, and scared also. Don't scream, don't leave the room; sit there. Try to just be present. I know this is hard, but you can do it. Remember this: Moms always love you; they are always worried something bad will happen to you. It is just part of what a mom does.)

Mom: Have you seen a doctor?

Jenny: No, I'm afraid.

Mom: Well... I guess I will call and schedule an appointment.

Jenny: Will you come with me, Mom? I need you with me. (Be prepared for Mom to say she doesn't want to go, or maybe other things that she may not mean at this time. She is in shock, but she still loves you.)

Mom: I am hurt and angry, but yes I will come with you.

MOM QUESTIONS

And how about some questions from mom about your daughter and birth control? Girls, your mother may have as many privacy concerns as you. See what conversations emerge from these Q&As.

Q: If I allow my daughter to start taking birth control pills, am I encouraging her to have sex at an earlier age?

A: No, you are not encouraging her to have sex, you are either encouraging her to be responsible, or you are treating a medical problem. I have yet to meet a girl to whom I have prescribed the pill who has said, "Now I can go find a guy to have sex with." On the other hand, I see many girls who are having sex without any protection from pregnancy or STDs, and getting into trouble. If your child is thinking of having sex it is reasonable to strongly encourage abstinence, but making it the forbidden fruit will not keep her from doing it. This is a time to talk to your daughter about the ramifications of having sex and to talk about what sex is.

It is also a time to encourage her to "own her actions" and teach her responsibility for her body and herself. If she needs to take the pill for a medical reason, it disturbs me that people would withhold medical treatment out of their own fears. I have had girls who have incapacitating cramps and everything has been tried with no great improvement, and yet, the parents will refuse the pill. Would you withhold other medical treatment?

A 15-year-old girl, Cecilia, was sent to my office for follow-up from the emergency room where she was seen for acute lower abdominal pain. The night before, she developed sudden pain on her lower left side. It became so intense that she was unable to stand up, completely doubled over. Her parents took her to the emergency room to be evaluated for appendicitis. After blood work and abdominal ultrasound, the doctor concluded the pain was related to an ovarian cyst. By the time she showed up at my office the next day she was feeling much better, barely taking any pain medication.

In taking her history, without her parents in the room, I discovered that the young woman was sexually active and was not using birth control. She was adamant that her parents not find out about her having sex. I told her that I would try not to be the one to tell them; however, since she was a minor, they could have access to her medical record. I discussed at length the risk that she was taking by having unprotected sex and tried to encourage her to change her behavior and to talk to her parents.

In our discussion she told me her parents would be very upset if they were to find out that she was not a virgin. I encouraged her to rethink having unprotected sex. For her ovarian cyst, birth control pills would be one of the best treatments. I explained to her what an ovarian cyst was and why birth control pills would help the cyst and protect her from pregnancy as well. I reassured her that I would not announce that she was sexually active, but she should reconsider her behavior.

Later, in discussing the plan for using oral contraceptives to treat this with Cecilia, both parents were present. They were very upset about the treatment option because they thought it would encourage her to have sex, but they understood the importance of helping her medically. For quite some time they wrestled with the

*notion that using birth control pills to treat medical problems does
not necessarily promote having sex. For them, the issue was not
resolved in one office visit, but the visit did serve as the impetus for
conversations between Cecilia and her parents.*

*Q: My daughter has severe cramps, and her health care provider
has recommended birth control pills. How safe is this treatment?*

A: In a healthy young girl with no significant medical history it
is very safe. The biggest risk is going to be the blood clot risk, which, in
a healthy ambulatory patient, is very unlikely. I always see first-time pill
users back in three months to evaluate how they are doing. At that visit,
her blood pressure and weight will be assessed. I will also make sure the
pill is achieving the goals for which it was prescribed. For instance, if it
was prescribed for cramps, I want to make sure her cramps are better.
Also, good patient education is the key to avoiding problems with birth
control pills.

*Q: My daughter is not sexually active but has a boyfriend.
Should I buy her condoms?*

A: Mother instincts are generally good. If you think your
daughter is in a relationship in which sexual activity is going on or
is inevitable, it is time to have a heart-to-heart talk with your child.
This also requires good listening skills on your part. Most parents do
not want their 16-year-old daughter having sex, but the main priority
should be your child's safety. This is not a time to say "I forbid you
to have sex," but to talk to her about what sex means and how it can
impact her both physically and emotionally. *After* you have talked to
her, and if you feel she is having sex or about to have sex, then—yes—
equip her to be safe. Let her know you may not agree with her decision,
but she and her safety are extremely important to you.

*Q: My daughter has been put on birth control pills for her
irregular cycles. What are the most common side effects when she starts
the pill?*

A: The most common side effect that occurs when anyone starts
birth control pills is irregular bleeding. This bleeding, which can be very

light spotting or heavier, more like a period, is called breakthrough bleeding. This happens less than 15% of the time and will generally stop after the first month or two of taking the pills, as long as you keep taking them regularly.

The second most common side effect is change in mood. Often, birth control improves moodiness and premenstrual symptoms, but on occasion the moodiness gets worse. The third most common side effect is nausea. It is very rare but does occur. If your daughter has nausea, it is important to take her pill at night so that when the blood level is high she is, hopefully, sleeping soundly. By the time she wakes up, the level of hormones has dropped so much that the nausea is often gone. Other symptoms are breast tenderness, headaches, skin changes, and rarely weight gain.

The most important part of starting the oral contraceptives is to continue to take them regularly even if she has some side effects. If the adverse symptoms seem to be more than you think they should be, contact the person who prescribed them and discuss the problem before just stopping them. Remember, there are many different pills to try. If one doesn't seem to agree with her, the next one she tries may be perfect.

Rita, a 13-year-old girl, was having very severe cramps and heavy bleeding. After discussing it with both her and her mother, I decided to start her on the pill to see if it would help with both the cramps and the bleeding. I gave her a pack of pills and she took her first dose that evening. About 2 o'clock in the morning she went into her mother's room complaining of nausea and then proceeded to vomit. The next night when she took the pill she didn't throw up, and each day her nausea was less and less. Now she is able to take the pill during the day without any nausea or other side effect. She says that the best part is that her periods are regular and mostly cramp free.

TABLE TALK

Table Talk Conversation on Follow-up Visit.

Mom: I asked you to finish your chores and you haven't yet.

Liz: (Starts crying and snaps) I told you that I would finish them.

Mom: I notice in the last six weeks, since you started your pills to regulate your cycles, you seem much more emotional.

Liz: You are not the only one who has noticed this. My friends say I am more touchy as well.

Mom: It may be time to call the nurse practitioner to see if we need to change your pill. She said that we had many options.

Q: I have found condoms in my daughter's purse. What should I do?

A: Well, first of all, I am grateful that if your daughter is sexually active she is protecting herself and her partner. If your daughter is not eighteen, then I would be concerned. The idea of sex being sacred and based on a very intimate relationship is too overwhelming for anyone under the age of eighteen.

I would find a time when I could be still and listen to my daughter. Whether that happens over a meal at the kitchen table or a long car drive is really up to you. It is important not to lecture your daughter. Let her know you are there to listen to her. Try to understand what she is experiencing right now.

There is another issue: I don't know how you found the condom. Did it fall out of the purse accidentally? Or were you searching her purse for other things? If you found it accidentally, then I would confess to her what happened and see how she reacts. If you are looking in her purse for other items, then I am assuming you have trust concerns or other worries that you are not confident she is being honest. If you are experiencing lack of trust with your daughter, then confrontation will do little good and may even make things worse. In this case, I would suggest seeking a professional counselor with whom you can talk. And please don't wait!

Q: My sixteen year old is having sex. What should I do?

A: It is much easier to prevent than to stop sexual behavior. If your sixteen-year-old is having sex, I think there is a break-down in communication between mom and daughter (unless you have told her that it is okay for her to have sex before the age of eighteen). Being a parent is difficult work, and no one tells us how to do it. I would encourage you to sit down with your daughter and discuss the consequences of her behavior. The first consequence is the concept of *sacro sex*. She is only sixteen, and the chances of this being a relationship that will last are small.

This relationship may prevent your daughter from developing her own passions or pursuing her education to the fullest extent possible. If she is intimately involved with a boy, how does she participate in after-school activities, or go out with other friends? When she is older will she resent being in such a serious relationship with a boy when she was sixteen, and not experimenting with other relationships?

Being in a serious relationship at the age of sixteen prevents one from exploring his or her own beliefs and being accountable for actions. If your daughter gets pregnant or contracts a sexually transmitted disease, she will be affected for the rest of her life. Most girls want a mom who will take a stance and tell them what the rules are. They want clear boundaries that they can bounce against but not break. They have an excuse not to take risky chances if they have a mom who says, "No, we don't engage in that behavior in our house."

Sit down with your daughter at a table. Don't lecture; just share your fears and concerns. Tell her you will help her with setting new limits in the relationship (girls are afraid of disappointing a boyfriend). Be there for her. Tell her all the areas she is good at. Help her find her natural gifts and passions. Most girls who become involved in serious relationships before the age of eighteen are doing it for popularity. Also, take time to examine whether you are vicariously living through your daughter.

If you (Mom) wanted to date more than you did in your youth, or be more popular then you were, please talk with a therapist about it. Whatever you do, don't pass your desire on to your daughter. Your daughter has so many opportunities. She doesn't need a steady boyfriend; she needs a mom who is 100% behind her in being the most educated and confident woman she can become.

Q: But what if she's embarrassed to talk with me?

A: Many girls are embarrassed to talk to their parents about sex. They may feel you will judge them or not be pleased with their behavior. This is a great time to show your daughter that you can be a good listener and that you love her first and foremost. You do not have to agree that sex is okay. I am supporting you with that. Tell your daughter how you feel. She wants to know even if she says she doesn't. Tell her you love her but explain to her that sex involves emotions, a relationship and being able to talk about the consequences of making love.

Most girls under the age of eighteen cannot manage a sexual relationship physically or emotionally as well as be active in school and excellent in academics. Talk, listen, and listen more. Your goal is not to settle the problem or erase her concern. Your goal is to be open to your daughter and to be available. If she sees she can trust you and that you won't judge her, but rather help her, she will open up more and more. Be on her side. She will need you.

Q: I want to talk to my daughter about sex but I was sexually abused. Should I mention this when I talk to her?

A: First of all, let me tell you I am sorry this happened to you. It is a challenge for all of us to change and grow into sexual women. Sexual abuse is such a violating act done to us and makes the process of becoming healthy sexual women even more difficult. I am glad you are sensitive to your daughter's needs and are asking for advice on what is and is not appropriate. If you have worked through the abuse and don't have "shame feelings," or feelings that it was in any way your fault, you are ready to talk about it with your daughter.

I also think it may be advantageous for your daughter to hear your story (provided she is over the age of fourteen). She will be able to see you as a strong woman and someone who made it through something we all hope we never have to go through. It will also help her to understand how bad things can happen to innocent people who aren't doing anything wrong. I would talk to her about how beautiful sexuality is, but only if a person is ready and both partners are equals in the decision. This would be a good time to explain to her that there are consequences you must be ready for before you become sexually active. The most important thing you could share with her would be that, even though this happened to you, you were able to go on and love another person and have a daughter. Our children need to know we wanted them and that the minute they entered life we were there with open arms.

Q: How do I talk to my daughter about sex and honestly answer her questions like "When did you first have sex?" when I'm promoting abstinence?

A: This is a good question, Mom. The first point I want to stress with you is I believe you know your daughter better than any other person in the world. If your daughter is mature enough and is asking honestly, I believe an honest answer is best. You may want to stress what the consequences were for you having sex at a young age. What do you wish you would have done differently? What do you wish your mom would have done differently so this would not have happened? Realize that not all personal information is meant to be shared all at once—your primary goal is to connect, support, and instruct.

Remember, your daughter is not you. You are raising her differently and she is influenced by a different society then you had. Mostly, remember that you are the most influential teacher your daughter has. What you tell her will have more of an impact then anyone else. Tell her how you feel. Talk with her about her choices and her options. Empower her with knowledge so she will understand why girls choose to have sex. *Sexuality is sacred.* We are very clear that there is no wise reason to have sex before the age of 18 years.

Your daughter is lucky, for this is a question only a reflective, caring mom would ask.

Q: With all of the availability of birth control, is teen pregnancy really a problem?

A: Yes, it is. The United States has the highest rate of teen pregnancy of all developed countries. Many of the educational programs are based on abstinence-only philosophy, but do not take into account the fact that the average age of onset of sexual activity is approximately 15 years of age. That is why we need to teach girls about natural urges and how to handle them. We need to tell them they are not mature enough to be having sex before 18, and let them know how to prevent pregnancy and infections if they are having sex. After the brain has time to mature, it is capable of more understanding of consequences. We need to set limits with our children, minimizing situations that put them at risk. Avoiding these conversations does not help, and the consequences can be tough to cope with. We need to talk with our children.

TABLE TALK IDEAS AND CONVERSATION STARTERS

Conversation starters on the subject of birth control, and some recommended activities.

For moms:

1. Did you hear about that popular T.V. star who got pregnant at age 16? What do you think about that?

2. I read that the average age of first intercourse is 15. Do you know anyone who is active, and are they using birth control?

3. If you were in a relationship and it was beginning to get physical, would you feel comfortable coming to me for birth control?

4. Even though I prefer abstinence, you know that your health and well-being are what I care about the most, right?

5. Are there any pregnant girls at your school?

For daughters:

1. Mom, what are your thoughts on birth control pills for cramps?

2. Did you know that we have two pregnant teenagers at our school?

3. If I wanted birth control, could I come and ask you for it?

4. My friend has an ovarian cyst and her health care provider put her on birth control pills. Have you heard of this, and why would it work?

5. Mom, I was reading an article about birth control pills and some of the different reasons they are used. Did you ever take birth control pills?

6. Could you have gone to *your mom* and asked her for birth control?

7. I heard at school that there is never a good medical reason to start taking the pill. What do you think?

> *The first step towards change is acceptance. Once you accept yourself, you open the door to change. That's all you have to do. Change is not something you do. It's something you allow.*
>
> *—Will Garcia*

CHAPTER 6

"I'm so fat!"

BODY IMAGE, EATING DISORDERS, AND PSYCHOLOGICAL HEALTH

L et's talk about our bodies, how we feel about them, how we treat them, and what this has to do with health and sexuality.

Let's take a look at some questions we often get around eating and body image: *Anorexia, bulimia, food obsessions.*

Q: My daughter has always been obsessed with her weight, but recently she has become even more stressed by the idea of becoming fat.

She doesn't eat with us like she did, and seems very emotional around food events. My friend told me she looks anorectic. What does this mean?

A: *Anorexia nervosa* is a psychological condition where individuals (usually girls) restrict food in order to lose weight. This behavior can get out of control and result in extreme weight loss.

Anorexia is a disease (the desire to starve yourself thin), and it will not go away without treatment. It is more severe than just getting thin or wanting to play sports. It is something that requires treatment. What you have to remember as a mother is that low self-esteem and feelings of helplessness can contribute to the problem.

Most people with anorexia have a distorted view of their body size, no matter how thin they are. People with anorexia are often unusually sensitive about being perceived as "fat" and are terrified of gaining weight. If your daughter has any of the following symptoms she should see a family physician within the next week. Remember, there can also be other causes of weight loss, such as thyroid disease or diabetes, and only her health care provider can determine this.

- ❏ Excessive weight loss in a short period of time.

- ❏ Continued dieting, although she is already very thin.

- ❏ Unusual interest in food or food rituals.

- ❏ Eating very slowly and very little, and counting the bites or cutting food into very small pieces.

- ❏ Obsession with exercise.

- ❏ She uses body weight as a primary measure of self-worth.

- ❏ Your daughter has an extreme dissatisfaction with body image.

- ❏ Your daughter's actual weight is less then 85% of her "healthy body weight." According to Federal guidelines, a Body Mass Index (BMI) less than 18 is "underweight" and more than 24 is "overweight," but BMI may be most accurate after a teen has completed her growth.

❏ Your daughter begins to withdraw from family and friends.

❏ Your daughter suffers from fainting, irregular heart rate, or seizures.

If these behaviors have been going on for more than two weeks, your daughter may have anorexia nervosa. She will need to be seen by her pediatrician as well as a psychotherapist. I would advise you to start with her pediatrician and then follow their advice as to what you should do in conjunction with that.

Q: What causes my daughter to become so upset with food, even willing to starve herself skinny?

A: It is not known what causes *anorexia nervosa*, but there are several factors at play. These include family dynamics and peer pressures. There has been some research in the field of chemical imbalances, which is why some medications may be helpful. The family genetics should also be considered, as well as longstanding emotional problems. The media is also not without blame. The media are full of images of the "ideal body" which leads girls often to set unrealistic and unattainable body shape and weight goals for themselves. Sports, too, can play a part in putting pressure on girls to stay thin. For example, gymnastics, ballet, ice-skating and other sports stress low body weight for the girls to be competitive. This is not to say that athletics are of themselves bad, but they can contribute to anorexia if the girl is predisposed.

Q: My daughter has been diagnosed with anorexia nervosa. Is it possible this will go away if I do nothing? I don't want to upset her with her friends knowing she is getting treatment for this disorder.

A: I understand that it may be embarrassing for your daughter to go to treatment. Or maybe you are embarrassed, as her mom, and don't want to put the whole family through this. Unfortunately, anorexia will not go away by itself. If untreated, this disorder may lead to serious health problems, sometimes including death. Severe restriction of food can have dangerous effects on the body, especially the heart, brain, and bones. The heart can actually weaken and serious heart problems can develop. The brain can shrink, causing changes in personality, and the bones can lose calcium which may make them weak and more likely to break. Taking supplements does not protect from malnutrition.

Anorexia is also associated with psychological disorders like depression and obsessive compulsive behaviors. There are other problems that may develop as a result of anorexia, including extreme sensitivity to cold, weak/brittle nails, a grayish appearance, hair loss, and growth of fine hair on the arms, face, shoulders, and back. Women with anorexia experience amenorrhea or the loss of menstrual periods. It is possible to die from anorexia nervosa. (Remember Karen Carpenter?)

Q: My daughter is getting treatment from her pediatrician for anorexia nervosa. How can we (as a family) help support her during this time?

A: The fact that you are asking this question makes me believe your daughter is in a loving, caring family. The first thing you should all do is educate yourselves about anorexia nervosa. Make sure your daughter knows that everyone is there for her, and cares and wants to help.

Don't pressure your daughter about eating, and try not to talk about weight or food. Be patient. This is a process; change takes a long time. The issues are always more complicated then just food. Be prepared as a family. Your daughter may think she is getting better than she is and may get angry or at times even refuse your help. A helpful place to begin is a web site for recovery from anorexia and bulimia: http://www.something-fishy.org.

*Q: My daughter has been caught twice now (by her little brother) throwing up after meals. I am concerned because, although she tells me it is nothing, she is losing weight. What should I do? When I talk to her she says it is "nothing." Is it possible it could be **bulimia**?*

A: This is *not a nothing*. This is *something*. I would start out by talking to your daughter. It is important that you ask when this started.

How frequently does it happen? Is she forcing it, or is she throwing up naturally? Your daughter may be exhibiting a form of anorexia called binge eating/purging. This is where the individual eats a large amount of food in a short period of time (binges) and then vomits or uses laxatives (purges). Most people with bulimia will maintain a normal or above normal weight by binging and purging, while people with anorexia have weight below normal.

It is important that you tell your daughter that you are concerned, then listen to her. Just listen. Don't criticize her but do validate how difficult it must be for her. Tell her you are on her side and that you want to help her. Schedule an appointment with your family doctor or pediatrician and go to the appointment with her. You will both need to become invested in the treatment. The pediatrician may suggest you also get a psychotherapist as well as a psychiatrist. Don't let this scare you.

Your daughter may also have a mental illness such as bi-polar disease. This disease often presents itself around the age of seventeen or eighteen. Addictions (such as increased food consumption or starving oneself) may be one of the first symptoms. The pediatrician or health care professional may suggest a dietician also. If they don't, it would be a good idea for you to request this service. Many times, it is not thought of, but a dietician can be the most important person you can have on your team.

Q: How do I know if my daughter has symptoms of Bulimia Nervosa or if she is just going through a "stage" where she wants to look pretty for a boy? My friends all say I am over-reacting because I am very concerned that I think she may be binging and then purging.

A: You are a wise mom to be concerned. You are also not over-reacting. You have reason to be concerned over your daughter's behaviors. Both girls and boys with bulimia seek out binge and purge episodes. They will eat a large quantity of food in a relatively short period of time (within a two-hour span) and then use behaviors such as taking a laxative or self-inducing vomiting because they feel overwhelmed in coping with their emotions. Or, they may unrealistically wish to punish themselves for something they feel they should be blamed. This can be in direct relation to how they feel about themselves, or how they feel over a particular event or series of events in their lives. Those suffering with bulimia may also have episodes of binging and purging to avoid feelings of anger, depression, stress or anxiety. Research suggests that for a percentage of sufferers, a genetic predisposition may play a role in sensitivity to develop bulimia in response to environmental factors. Most people who have bulimia are aware they have an eating disorder.

Q: So what should I look for in Bulimia?

A: Look for the following:

- ❏ Recurring episodes of rapid food consumption followed by tremendous guilt and purging (laxatives, self-induced vomiting, compulsive exercise)

- ❏ A feeling of lacking control over her eating behaviors.

- ❏ Regularly engaging in strict diet plans and exercise.

- ❏ Abusing laxatives, diuretics, and or diet pills.

- ❏ A persistent concern of her body image, as evidenced in comments, compulsions, questions.

Both bulimia and anorexia are serious. There is a common risk of a history of sexual, physical and/or emotional abuse in both illnesses, and a strong connection in some people between eating disorders and clinical depression. A physician will know how to help you decide which of these, if any, are possible and how best to get help for your daughter. The main point is, *do not ignore it*. It will not go away. Talk with your daughter and reassure her that you will help her. You don't have to have all the answers, but as long as your daughter feels like you will help her and she will not be alone and overwhelmed by her disease, she can heal.

I received a call from a plastic surgeon. Apparently he had a young woman (age fifteen) who came to see him for breast implants. I was startled because what fifteen year old can even drive? How did this young woman even get to the plastic surgeon?

You have probably already guessed. Her mother, of course, brought her in.

The reason I was called in was because the mother became irate when the surgeon told her that he would NOT put breast implants in a girl who was only fifteen. Upon my meeting the young girl I almost cried. What kind of a mother would acquiesce to this type of surgery and even promote it for her own daughter? The girl told me she felt badly about her small breasts and she wanted bigger ones so others would not comment on them. She also felt like she would "fit in" with bigger breasts. I was blown away. I talked to the mother. The mother said she felt her daughter should be able to have the implants so she could be popular and wear the clothes that would look more attractive on her. WHAT WAS HER MOTHER THINKING? I wanted to report her to Children's Protective Services! I think this is a form of abuse. The daughter had nothing wrong with her. She was small and thin, but it was obvious she was not fully grown. Her breasts fit her.

I went on to tell the mother that she should focus on her own breasts and not her daughter's. I told her that her daughter needed a mother to listen to her and support her with good sound advice. Without knowing it (or maybe she did) this mother was telling this daughter that she was not okay. She was giving her permission to do something that could be harmful to her and her health.

I will tell you and any mother reading this book: your child does not need plastic surgery to "fit in" or be more popular. She needs a mother who will validate her beauty and support her and guide her into finding her own passions. A mother should be there to remind the child how wonderful she is. How special she is, and also to point out her areas of weakness when that applies. If your daughter has a burn or a mark that is causing her stress or unwelcome remarks from peers, that is something else. But if she wants bigger breasts, a better nose, or anything else involving pure cosmetic surgery, tell her that being under the age of eighteen is not a good time to try and make decisions that are irreversible. Don't ever promote surgery for your daughter when it isn't necessary. I believe this mother and anyone like her may have severe emotional issues that she never worked through for herself. It saddens me to think she would use her daughter to work through the old junk in her own trunk. A psychologist would be a more helpful professional for her to visit... not a plastic surgeon.

TABLE TALK

Food, Eating, and Self-Image Here are some suggestions of ways you may want to bring up the subject with your daughter. You know your daughter best, so feel free to look at these suggestions and then make your own best attempt.

Attempt this talk at a time when you are not rushed and neither of you is feeling irritable. Ask your daughter to schedule a time to talk. When the two of you are ready, sit down with her and start the conversation by telling her how you can empathize with some of the pressure she may feel in school, making grades, relationships, and just being a teenager. Tell her some of the times you remember being stressed out and what you tried to do to control these feelings. Then tell her how concerned you are with her and her apparent feelings in regards to food. The conversation may look like this:

Mom (Ellen); Daughter (Jennifer)

Ellen: Jennifer, I am wondering ... do you have stress in your life? What can I do to help you alleviate some of the stress you have right now. I can see you are trying so hard with homework, school, relationships, sport. I don't know how you do it.

Jennifer: Thanks Mom, but I have it under control. I just worry so much, and I feel like everything is out of control. I feel overwhelmed sometimes.

Ellen: Yes, I remember that time in my own life. I was so stupid at times, and I felt so alone. I never felt like I could go to my mom and talk to her.

Jennifer: You felt stupid? I can't imagine you ever felt that way.

Ellen: Many times. I would try things and then feel guilty and wish I hadn't. I would beat myself up and many times I didn't like myself.

Jennifer: Yeah, I feel that way sometimes too, Mom. The only thing I can control is my food. I guess I am doing that. I get angry because you make it a big deal, and it is the only thing I feel like I have control over.

Ellen: I am just worried you will get sick. I don't think the way you are dealing with food is healthy. I want to help you, but I don't know how.

Jennifer: I will be okay.

Ellen: I love you, Jennifer. You are everything to me. How about if we both go to see a counselor together? We can both learn about managing this, and maybe together we can support each other.

Jennifer: Well okay, but only once.

Ellen: How about if we talk to the counselor and then see what they suggest? We will take it one day at a time, okay? I only want what is best for you.

Jennifer: Okay, Mom.

Q: I suspect my daughter may be taking drugs. What should I do?

A: This is every parent's worst nightmare, and the first thing you must remember is this is not a time to react — this is a time to respond. But you do not want to act before you think things over carefully, and become fully aware of what is happening. You will need to write down how she has changed. Why do you suspect it? Have you found any evidence? What do her teachers say? How are her grades? Does she have different friends then she did before? Is she disrespectful of you?

Is she lying? Is she breaking the law by using illegal drugs? Are there prescription drugs in your medicine cabinet? The number one form of drug abuse is now prescription drugs available in the house.

As you start doing your homework and writing things down, the next thing to do is seek an adolescent counselor. You may ask friends if they have names of good therapists. You can also ask the school and speak to their counselor on staff. Once you have a therapist established, you will have to talk with your daughter. It is important that you tell her you are concerned with her behavior and that you love her. From here, you will have to get tough. You will have to tell her that you believe she needs to attend counseling with you. Make sure the therapist knows the whole family is supporting your daughter. This is very important, as the therapist most likely will want to see the whole family. If your daughter is indeed addicted to a substance, she will be angry and defensive. Remember, the drug is in control, and this person is not your daughter anymore. This person is your daughter under the influence of a drug. She is not the same person, and you must remain clear about this. You will have more strength to do what you need to do if you keep this in the back of your mind. It is very scary, but you can turn things around. If you do nothing, things will only get worse. There are help lines suggested in the back of the book. We are all with you. Good luck.

Q: I think my daughter is being bullied. What can I do to help?

A: When I was a child and young adolescent, I knew kids who were bullied. I remember that not a lot was done on the family level or school level. These girls grew up as we all did. I have had the opportunity to watch them and what happened in their life. Most of them ended up having low self-esteem and became addicted to food, alcohol or other unhealthy vices. Research has shown that bullying is serious business. It needs to be taken very seriously. As a mother, these are the steps you must take when your daughter confides that she is being bullied. The steps involve looking at your own mentoring, and seeing how you measure up as a good role model.

Acknowledge your role of teasing and gossiping in your own life. Has she watched you do this? Is she learning to do what you do? Studies have shown that teachers who were bullied actually are the worst bullies. If you gossip (mean) or tease your child will certainly act that out. Turn off the television if it features T.V. gossip shows.

Never tell your daughter to ignore the teasing. We know it will not go away.

Begin working on your daughter's tone of voice so she can sound confident and purposeful in her speech.

Teach your daughter how to walk confidently. Shoulders back, a sure walk, and a look that she means business.

Your goal at first will be for her to know that the two of you are a team. If your daughter says this is not working and begins showing signs of being afraid to go to school, or if she cannot concentrate in school or begins to voice feeling powerless or trapped, it is time to get the school authorities involved. Tell your daughter that you will not make the situation worse and that you will be with her in dealing with this. Talk to the school principal by making an appointment. The principal can guide you and your daughter at that point. Schools have a NO BULLY POLICY because they know the danger of bullying. They will not tolerate it. Congratulate your daughter on speaking up. That is a bold and wise decision. It is another great opportunity for you to model strong behavior and what being a confident woman looks like for your daughter.

Q: I understand that "bully behavior" is not tolerated in schools. Now my daughter has told me that she is being bullied on the computer. Is this something new? What can I do to help?

A: The type of bullying you are speaking of is called *cyberbullying*. Nintey percent of middle school students have had their feelings hurt on line.

Forty percent have visited a Web site bashing another student.

40% have had their passwords stolen and changed by a bully (who then locked them out of their own account or sent communications posing as them).

Only 15% of parents polled knew what cyberbullying was.[4]

Cyberbullies use e-mail, instant messages (IMs), cell phones, text messages, photos, videos and social networking sites to humiliate and threaten others. This is an example: a student may use her cell-phone to take a picture of a classmate changing clothes after gym, then uploads it onto her computer and forwards it to friends along with cruel commentary. What makes cyberbullying so easy and tempting is the anonymity the Web provides, along with a potentially huge audience.

Often, if you think you can be anonymous, there's no fear of detection. Even if you identify yourself, you don't see people's reaction or realize you have gone too far. For the victim, cyberbullying can be especially damaging because it's so pervasive. Your child may get IMs saying that everyone hates her and/ or she should watch her back. She may never know who really is behind it. This leads to problems with focus and an inability to concentrate while at school. Your daughter may become paranoid and anxious.

If you think your daughter is doing the cyberbullying, advise your daughter to be the same person online as she is in real life. If she wouldn't say something to someone when they were with her, she shouldn't write it and send it on line. Don't be intimidated by technology. Sit down with your daughter and go through her web sites like My Space, You Tube and Facebook. If you discover that your child has targeted someone, take away the weapon, the computer or cell phone, and make her earn it back. Laws are being set up now to make cyberbullying follow the same guidelines as other types of bullying. Until those laws are solid and in place, make sure you understand where your daughter goes in cyberspace and to whom she is talking. If she tells you there is a problem, believe her. *There is a problem.*

One of the first patients I ever saw at Houston Child Guidance was a young girl who was "acting out" terribly. She was placed in this alternative school because the public school could not handle her behavior. She was very angry, overweight, and basically had no friends and kept repeating that she did not want any. She had scars all over her arms where she had cut herself to watch herself bleed. She had dyed her hair raven black. She was so continuously sad it hurt me just to see her. One day I asked her to come to my office after she was done with her school work. When she came in to see me, we talked for a long while. I got to know her name, her history, and her own story about why she was at Houston Child Guidance.

She related to me that she had been the victim of terrible bullying since four years old. She said her parents never took her seriously and told her to "handle it." Erica was so terrified; she couldn't sleep at night and suffered from terrible stomach pain. The pain went on year after year. Finally, at the ripe old age of 10 years, she tried to kill herself. This got the attention of all those around her except her parents. As I listened to Erica, my heart went out to her. What a sad young girl, who had learned to take matters into her own hands and fight back. Her defiance and determination got her kicked out of school and placed in Houston Child Guidance, but it also kept her alive. Her parents missed a great opportunity to support and love Erica. I don't know what happened to Erica, but I am assuming it was not a happy ending.

Please, if your daughter tells you that she is being bullied, believe her. Jump in and support her. Alert the school and authorities if you need to. Do not think it will go away by itself. Your daughter needs your help!

Q: Is there a connection between bullying and sexual behaviors?

A: Bullying is an aggressive action of violence toward someone else. It is like other violent behaviors in the way that it uses threats, obscenity or harassment. It can involve stalking, or hate crimes, or it may involve pornography. When sex is not kept sacred, it may have some of these same patterns. Bully behavior is a learned behavior. Usually the bully grew up with bullies or was bullied at another time in their life. It is unhealthy, it is risky, and it is disrespectful of others. Since violence and extortion may be part of bullying, you may see an increase in sexual acting out among bullies.

Q: What do I do if I discover that my daughter is sending catty messages, or that she is bullying others?

A: This question is so heartbreaking and, unfortunately, we are seeing more of it in the schools and everywhere. Girls are twice as likely as boys to be victims and perpetrators of cyberbullying. It is important for you as her mom to understand cyberbullying can occur any time of the day or night. Cyberbullying messages and images can be distributed quickly to a very wide audience. It may be almost impossible to track down or trace the cyberbully. Here are some things you can do to prevent and stop your daughter from cyberbullying. If it has gone too far, I suggest you talk with her about your seriousness in stopping it. Both you and she should attend a support group for cyberbullying. Your last option is to contact your local police and solicit their help with this matter. *This is very serious; do not drop it.*

1. Keep your home computers in easily viewable places, such as a family room or kitchen.

2. Talk to your daughter specifically about cyberbullying, on-line activities or anything she is involved in.

3. Encourage her to tell you about anyone else who may be involved in the cyberbullying (there is usually an extensive network working together against one or two children).

4. Explain to her that cyberbullying is harmful and unacceptable behavior. Make it clear to her there will be consequences enforced by you if she does not follow your family rules.

5. This may be the most difficult part. Although we must respect the privacy of our daughters, we must also be concerned with their safety as well as the safety of other children. These concerns may override privacy concerns. Tell your daughter you may review her on-

line communications if you believe there is reason to be concerned. Remember, your daughter will not be pleased with this, but you are her mom and safety for her is your primary concern.

Q: My mom says that teens are more stressed out today than before. Is that true? Why??

A: The more technologically adept we become, the more stress we seem to accumulate. It is ironic that we develop technologies to make tasks easier, but with each of these advancements, tasks also become more involved. More is expected of teens as we develop more areas of study. The world is becoming smaller and with that we are all becoming a bit more stressed.

One of the problems is that everyone seems to be so busy that we don't slow down for the good ol' visits like we use to. When is the last time you made cookies with your daughter and sat at the kitchen table with tea and cookies? Or when is the last time you took your daughter for a walk? These times build more than just communication. They teach your daughter to take time, talk and decompress. Do any of us know healthy ways of dealing with stress? Do we teach our daughters to breathe or smell lavender in the same way we grill them on their algebra questions?

Probably not, because we feel that their future is more secure if they know their algebra. Nothing could be further from the truth. Research shows that the most successful people in the world have great coping skills. Take time, listen to soft music, teach your daughter about keeping a journal, taking a bubble bath, having tea, and sometimes just sitting and doing nothing. You will be teaching her how to cope with life. None of us can avoid stress.

Q: How can I help my teen experience less stress, more success?

A: You do not determine your daughter's stress level. Some girls are anxious and tightly wired at birth. Others are so laid back you wish you could light a fire underneath them. It is neither your fault nor to your credit whatever kind of child you have. They are a spark of the stars, and individual in their own right. But you do have a lot of influence on how they handle stress. I have two daughters. The first one is very tightly wired and expresses her emotions like a verbal robot. I like to get away from her verbal recount of how she feels, as she is very aware of how she feels at all times. When she gets stressed, the whole house is aware of it, as she is verbally outraged. My other daughter appears to be very laid back. She is not, though. She bites her fingernails, grinds her teeth at night, and suffers from feeling depressed from time to time because she cannot express how she feels with words. You may identify with some of this and, therefore, I have written some of my favorite de-stressors for you.

These may help, and maybe as you visit with your daughter she can come up with a list of her own ideas of how to lower her stress. Don't be surprised if it is time away from the family. Teens seem to need a lot of time alone to think about issues. Respect their need for time alone.

Table Talk

Ideas for De-Stressors. *How about some of these de-stressors, from Debbie and her mom?*

Mom: What works for me is a hot bubble bath.

Debbie: For me .... calming music.

Mom: Or lavender spray on pillows.

Debbie: I'd go for a comedy that makes me laugh.

Mom: Learning to breathe through my belly; don't for get about that one.

Debbie: Better yet, a massage.

Mom: Or a pedicure or manicure?

Debbie: Some of your home-made chicken soup.

Mom: And of course, time alone with you.

Debbie: Exercise (even walking, hiking, or taking a class).

Mom: I'd settle for going to the park and sketching trees.

Debbie: Or journaling.

Mom: Yeah, and then there are comfort foods.

Q: Do you have some recommendations on healthy living, especially healthy living for Cheeto®-loving mom and daughter?

A: Establishing a healthy lifestyle at a young age is a one of the best ways to ensure healthy living as an adult. Many factors influence healthy living, including diet and exercise, adequate sleep habits, stress reduction, personal connections, and safety.

Q: Are there tips for healthy eating?

A: Here's our list of "DO's":

❏ Eat breakfast everyday. If you prefer, try one of the many available protein drinks that are easy to consume on the run.

❏ Eat three meals a day and snacks in between.

❏ Fruits and veggies make great snacks.

❏ Eat foods high in fiber, such as whole grains.

❏ Be involved in planning meals.

❏ Stay well hydrated.

❏ Keep the food pyramid in mind in planning your meals and snacks.

Q: But before the age of 17, it doesn't really matter what I eat, right? There's nothing I really need to avoid. That's just for old moms, right?

A: DON'Ts for healthy eating, at any age:

- ❏ **Avoid** foods high in sugar such as juices and candy

- ❏ Limit caffeine intake

- ❏ Avoid high fat foods such as whole milk and fried foods

- ❏ Don't eat frequently at fast food restaurants, and don't get big sizes just because they offer it or because it is "a good deal."

- ❏ Don't keep unhealthy snacks around the house.

- ❏ Don't skip meals, especially breakfast, for you are breaking an overnight fast.

- ❏ Don't be afraid to try new and different foods.

Q: What about exercise?

A: Exercise is an important habit that should be done throughout your life. It can start in early childhood through play, riding bikes, participating in team sports such as soccer, or dance, or at a minimum, exercise that gets your heart rate up. As children reach adolescence, it is important to make exercise part of their life, even if they become less active in team sports or dance. At a minimum, exercise that gets their heart rate up should be done at least three days a week for at least 30 minutes. Some ideas on ways to achieve this goal are:

- ❏ Mothers and daughters go to the gym.

- ❏ Decide to support a good cause by running in fund raising races together.

- ❏ Encourage friends to exercise together.

- ❏ Schedule exercise just as you would schedule any other appointment.

❏ Take a dance class together.

❏ Start bike riding.

❏ Take up roller blading.

Q: What about sleep? How many hours should my daughter sleep?

A: Although the typical teen needs approximately 8-9 hours of sleep per night, fewer than 25% of teens get adequate sleep. Sleep deprivation several nights in a row, and then trying catch up by sleeping all day on the weekend, does not make up for sleep that is missed. Not getting enough sleep can interfere with the ability to concentrate, make you more accident prone, and can decrease you immune system, causing you to be more prone to illness. Too little sleep can affect your mental health and lead to depression.

There are a number of things you can do to ensure adequate sleep. Have a bed time and stick to it as much as possible. Limit activities that interfere with the ability to get enough sleep. Don't have the mind set that sleeping all day will make up for sleep that you have missed. Stay organized so that it is easy for you to get enough sleep.

Q: What do I do if I can't get to sleep? My brain keeps racing, and I obsess over my grades, my friends, and my boyfriend. I don't want to bother my mom, because I know she can't do anything about it.

A: This is a great question! We all sometimes have trouble falling asleep and letting go of things that happened during the day. One of the easiest ways to stop this behavior and also learn a lot about yourself is to keep a pad of paper with a pencil next to your bed. *Every* time you have a thought, write it down. The next day you can go over everything that you have written. This is a great exercise, and I promise the list will get smaller and smaller with each night you do it. Try it for at least two weeks. The great thing is that you can set a time the next day to review your list with your mom and get her advice when you are both rested.

Q: My daughter is a night-owl. She likes to sleep all day and stay up all night. Should I worry about it?

A: This may be a problem if she has after school activities and becomes tired. I have a rule at my home with my daughters. The first rule is no phone calls after 10:30 p.m. and the Internet (in an openly viewed part of our home) until 10p.m. for homework only. This seemed to help with my night owls.

*Q: What do I do if I'm mad at my mom, because she makes me **more** stressed?*

A: This is really a good question, and I want to reassure you that you and many girls say this. Try to engage your mom at a time when you are both rested and can have some time to just visit. Plan a walk, or go to a coffee shop. Tell her exactly what you asked here. But begin it by saying something like: "Mom, I know you love me, but sometimes you stress me out because of the way you _____ (fill this in)." You may want to write this down so you have a couple of things planned to say. If you start the conversation by telling her she is important to you, and reassuring her that you love her, she will be more apt to really listen and try to help. *Remember… no one loves you like your mom.* We cannot help it that sometimes we naturally annoy our daughters.

Q: I hear that so many of my daughter's friends are on antidepressants. Is depression more common among teenagers now than it used to be?

A: I appreciate your question. My daughter's whole sophomore class seemed to be on antidepressants or medication for attention deficit disorder with or without hyperactivity. I sometimes would question their diagnoses. I think that sometimes this may be a combination of ineffective parenting in the early years and lack of structure. I do think children today are exposed to many stressors, although I am not convinced it was more than when I was a teenager. I think the most dramatic change has been that both parents work outside the home and there seems to be less communication between parents. I believe parents expect the schools to parent more, which will never be as effective as parents' efforts. This being said, I do see depression among young women. I think the way you can help as a parent is to keep the lines of communication open. Encourage your daughter to journal and write down her feelings. Often, girls feel so intensely that they act dramatic and vent to their parents with arguments as the end result. If you can tell your daughter that her feelings are important but that she must learn how to express them constructively, she will succeed in channeling her feelings of stress, sadness, and depression into more healthy behaviors (for example, some of the best artists in high school are the girls whose parents have taught them to express their sadness feelings through art).

Q: How do I know if I'm depressed?

A: Teenage depression and anxiety are not limited to these symptoms, but these are some of the more common ones. It is important to remember that everyone gets depressed and anxious at times. But you may want to seek attention from a mental health provider if it continues in excess of two weeks with no change.

❑ Weight loss.

❑ Tired most of the time.

❑ Irritability.

❑ Loss of pleasure in events that used to bring a sense of joy.

❑ Crying or extreme moodiness.

❑ Anger outburst that becomes more frequent.

❑ Meltdowns that are brought about with little or no provocation.

❑ Isolation.

❑ Not wanting to talk to mom, sister, or other family members.

❑ Loss of friends or not going to social gatherings.

❏ Grades that begin declining.

❏ Shaking of hands, or stuttering.

❏ No future goals or curiosity.

Q: Do you have some ideas for stress reduction?

A: Here are some thoughts to try. Make it a mother-daughter experiment.

Listen reflectively. Ask what's wrong. Listen calmly and non-judgmentally, allowing your daughter to express her opinions. Refrain from offering advice. Get the whole story by asking questions like, "And then what happened?" Or ask her "how did that make you feel"?

Notice out loud. Casually observe your child's feelings. Say something like, "It seems like you're still frustrated about the outcome of that problem." Rather than sounding accusatory, you're letting your child know you're interested in hearing more.

Comment on your daughter's feelings. Show her that you understand and care by saying something like, "That must have been upsetting." This can help your daughter feel more connected to you.

Provide emotional support. Don't criticize or belittle your daughter's stressful feelings, even if they appear trivial. Remember that teens don't have the perspective that we adults do. Some issues—especially those relating to relationships and body image—are extremely important to them.

Provide realistic expectations. While we all want our daughters to get good grades, realize that if your child struggles with a subject like math or foreign language, a lower grade may be a real achievement for her if she is making her best effort. Celebrate your daughter's successes and let her know you're proud of her. Remind your daughter that occasionally feeling stressed is normal; that everyone feels angry or scared sometimes. You may share with her how you feel stress before a presentation or some other anxiety-provoking event.

Provide structure, stability and predictability. Prepare your daughter for a potentially stressful situation like a doctor or dentist appointment. Make sure your daughter understands your rules and routines, and stick with them. If she breaks a rule, follow through with the consequences. Don't bend rules or change consequences due to stressful events. It is wiser to prepare her for the upcoming event so she can prepare herself and know what to expect from you. Your daughter needs boundaries and expectations. This will actually help lower her stress.

Model positive coping skills. If you practice good problem-solving and coping skills — like exercising, laughing or taking a break to reduce your own stress level — your child will learn from you. Don't criticize yourself or your daughter—ever.

Help your child brainstorm a solution. Suggest activities that will help your daughter feel better now while also solving the problem. Ask your daughter for ideas of ways to solve the problems. Praise her when she comes up with creative solutions to her own problems. This will help build her confidence and self esteem.

Be organized. Early on, teach your daughter good organizational and time-management skills. This will make homework more manageable and less overwhelming, giving her more time to relax. A good way to start this is to have her pick out what she will wear to school the night before, and if she is packing a lunch, make sure she plans healthy foods.

Just be there. Even if your daughter doesn't feel like talking, she will still appreciate your presence. Being available to take a walk or watch a movie together shows you care about her.

Get professional help. If your daughter's behavior changes dramatically, she exhibits serious anxiety or she's having trouble functioning at home or school, ask your doctor to refer you to a mental health specialist.

Exercise and eat regularly. Exercise releases hormones in our bodies, which actually decrease our stress level.

Take a break. The relaxation response is our body's natural antidote to stress. Simple breathing exercises and muscle relaxation techniques can help trigger that response. For example ,"breathe" with your daughter. It is simple to do. Count one, two, three, four, five on the intake breath. Then together breathe out slowly to the count of eight. If you laugh together, it is okay. Breathing slowly and deeply decreases the heart rate and lowers the blood pressure. Both of these help relax your body.

Encourage meditation, prayer, relaxation tapes, or yoga. And make sure your daughter takes the time to do something she enjoys, like listening to music, watching TV, reading a book or writing in a journal when she is feeling overwhelmed or stressed.

Get support. Encourage your daughter to hang out with friends who help her cope in a positive way. Maybe you can have a backyard fire and roast marshmallows for celebrating "I am stressed day"! Your daughter will learn that taking a "mental health break" is fun and part of taking care of herself.

Be realistic. Assure your daughter that it's okay for her not to be perfect and encourage her to feel good about her accomplishments, even if they're not perfect

Don't over-schedule. If your child is feeling overwhelmed, make sure she concentrates on just the activities that really interest her and lets go of the others. Don't be afraid to step in here, Mom. Your daughter at times will get involved with too many activities. It may be difficult for you because you will have to be firm and say "NO." Remember, your job is to be her mom, and always do what is in your daughter's best interests. Your daughter may be angry with you for not letting her do what she wants. She even may be very dramatic. But you have the experience and knowledge to know what is best for her even though she may not agree.

Solve the little problems. Your daughter will gain a sense of control by solving everyday problems. Have her identify the problem, figure out options and take action toward a solution. One of the greatest ways of dealing with stress is to break the causes into smaller parts and handle each part one at a time.

Encourage your daughter to develop assertiveness. Teach your daughter to express her feelings politely but firmly. Have her practice saying, "I feel angry when you yell at me," or "Please stop yelling." This is difficult for many girls, but learning to express themselves calmly and not emotionally will save them from developing potential addictive behaviors in the future. Many obese people deal with emotions by eating. They never learned to say how they feel, so they eat their emotions rather then express them.

As difficult as it is to watch your daughter suffer through her everyday frustrations and stresses, you can't solve all of her problems. Nor should you try. But you can teach her to calmly manage her stress by focusing on coping skills and problem-solving techniques. Patience and understanding is most important for our daughters as well as their moms. Remember: growing up is a process, and you are building a foundation for generations to come.

> *Donna, a patient of mine, came into the office for a routine exam. I noticed that she was on medication for attention deficit disorder and also taking an antidepressant. I questioned the patient and her mother about this, and she proceeded to tell me the history. Donna seemed healthy and happy. I was told that she was doing well in school. Her mom told me that she was an early reader and always had been in the gifted classes. In second grade she began having a hard time finishing her work, and her teacher wrote it off as being lazy or unable to concentrate. Her mom took her for educational testing and she was found to have a high IQ and no definite signs of ADD or a learning disability. At this time she also developed a facial tic.*
>
> *Her teachers and her pediatrician told them to break things into smaller tasks and not pressure her. From that point until 6th grade, she was an A/B student. Nonetheless, at every school conference the teachers would tell the parents that if she would just work a bit harder she would be a straight A student. As she proceeded through middle school her grades were up and down, and she and her mother fought all of the time about grades. At the beginning of 8th grade her grades plummeted and she began having anxiety attacks.*

Her parents again had educational and psychological testing done. The testing revealed anxiety/depression, as well as some ADD tendencies. At first she was placed on medication for her anxiety and depression and she began to feel better, but she was still struggling with grades. She then was placed on a stimulant for ADD. Her mom describes it as though a light switch was turned on. Her grades came back up and her daughter was much happier. The relationship between the mother and daughter also improved, because the mom had a better idea of her daughter's need. Donna's grades continued to improve but there were occasional bumps in the road. Both the mom and Donna could recognize when she was overwhelmed and could begin to help Donna cope. Donna also realized how much support her mom could be. Mom commented that even though they found the medication to be helpful to her daughter after years of struggling, more importantly it allowed mother to approach her daughter from a different angle. It was easier to replace the lengthy lectures with into-the-night conversations.

Q: Do you have any thoughts on family, friends and raising a daughter in a spirit of community?

A: This book talks a lot about keeping relationships sacred. Just as sexuality is sacred, so are relationships within the family and among friends. Healthy daughters are born to parents who regard their family in a respectful and "sacred manner."

In fact, here are some thoughts for both moms and daughters together:

Teach your daughter to become responsible for her own emotional life. Your daughter needs to learn that no one should make her feel in a particular way. The only person who should have control over how she feels is herself. If your daughter isn't getting the results she wants, teach her that maybe it is her way of acting and behaving that is getting in her way. Feelings are never right or wrong; they just are. Our behavior, on the other hand, may be judged and usually is by others. The sooner your daughter learns that she is not a victim, but that she is an active participant in her life, the better.

At times when you are feeling sorry for yourself reassure your mom that you aren't turning into a "Victim" (we worry about this). Tell her you just need a little "pity party." Get mom involved by making a cake and serving ice cream. It is a good idea to feel sorry for yourself sometimes; just don't get caught up in it and don't let it last longer then one evening.

Teach your daughter that healthy relationships are based on equality. When one person in the family or among friends criticizes, demeans, or asserts authority over another, it may temporarily improve the self-esteem of one by lowering another's. This is always a false sense of power though. Relationships must be based on mutual respect so that everyone can be free to create the best for the good of all. Think of your best friends. One of my dearest friends, the coauthor of this book, is a good example. I feel like "home" with her. When I am around her, I feel her respect and good will, and therefore we can both create. That creativity is the energy behind this book.

Teach your mom by telling her when she says something that makes you feel good or special. Tell her when you observe her doing something that makes one of your friends or neighbors feel special.

Teach your daughter to say what she needs or feels. The key is not to silence your daughter. The key is to guide her to express herself in a way that ensures that she can be heard and understood. This means communicating in a polite but assertive manner so her needs won't be made fun of or ridiculed. You are helping to raise a potential leader or mother for the next generation. Her ability to communicate her needs will allow her to help and mentor others in her community and family.

When you tell your mom what you need or feel, try not to scream it or cry. Your mom is learning too. She is worried if she is being a good mom for you. Don't forget to reassure her once in awhile about what a good mom she is.

Demonstrate your appreciation for your daughter and others in your community and family. Remember your daughter is watching you. If she sees you telling and showing people that they add value to your life, she will understand how important it is. We show love and support for others when we identify within others what we share in common with them. Peace is taught; the time is now.

If you have a good idea or a solution to a family problem, be sure to suggest it to your mom. Your mom thinks she has to have most of the solutions, but show her that sometimes you will think of great ideas too! If you don't share them, she will never know. Give your mom a little slack, and let her know what a genius she is raising from time to time.

For both moms and daughters, remember, please, that life is short. Don't waste your time being angry at each other. Talk. Talk at the table. Anger is fleeting; love is forever!

CHAPTER 7

"Becoming the Person I Want to Be"

NURTURING YOUR PASSIONS AND GIFTS

I remember bringing each of my daughters home from the hospital; my husband carrying all of the baby stuff and me carrying the most precious gift we could have ever imagined. My head was full of dreams, and my husband's thoughts were on protecting her and keeping her from harm. I knew what I wanted her to be; my husband just knew what she was going to be. It's difficult to recount how much we changed our visions as both my children began to talk and tell us what they would and would not be. Frequently, we found ourselves resisting their preferred directions, and trying to guide them into what we continued to want. What a mistake this would have been to keep doing so.

Our society continually tries to tell women what they should be: more beautiful, perhaps more thin, more engaging, and more receptive to others' needs. We have forgotten that these girls are the potential leaders and mothers of the next generation, and they need to know that they don't have to fulfill anyone's expectations other than their own.

Mothers must get behind their daughters and help them to make a difference. Listen to them, guide them, and don't try to make them popular. Support them so they can become what they are destined to be.

> *I remember my heart falling as I encouraged my first daughter to ice skate. I wanted a daughter who could dance and skate. She was small and had the perfect body for this sport. However, when I spent tons of money for classes and outfits only to find out that she hated it, I had to give up this dream. She preferred catching bugs. She had a natural gift and seemed to understand them. This passion grew to a love for all creatures. She majored in biology at the University of Texas, graduated, and is now a high school teacher for Advanced Placement in biology. She remembers how I tried to guide her into things she did not like. She was also blessed with a strong will — we used to fight a lot. I was lucky she did not give up her dreams for mine.*

Young adolescent girls don't need a boyfriend. They need a strong family, a dad who teaches them what a good man is and does, and a mother who is brave enough to make individual strides to be her own person. A daughter does not want you to be her friend. She wants you to be her mom.

Young women must understand their bodies, their sexuality, and their own passions and gifts. If a young woman is knowledgeable about sexuality, she will understand the consequences of having sex for the wrong reasons, and how wonderful it can be at the right time and for the right reasons. No woman benefits from having sex before she is involved with an intimate partner and before she is eighteen. She also needs to know how to protect her health when she does decide to have intimate contact and sex. Sexuality is sacred and not to be entered lightly. I want women to understand themselves fully before they try to please another person. I want girls to have the freedom to be all they can be before they worry about relationships with boys.

As moms, we can do better then we have in the past. We can expose our daughters to many activities while they are with us, so if they make mistakes in finding their way, we can guide and support them. Get behind me: be a mom; be a mentor. Be the kind of woman you desire, so your daughter will see that she is also free to be herself.

I have a psychology degree and a theology degree. One of the gifts I learned while studying theology is that we are all connected. Perhaps in more ways then we ever knew. I don't think it is wise to rigidly teach your child to be of a certain faith if it means she cannot support and care for persons of other faiths. After all, as Dr. Wayne Dyer suggests in his book *The Power of Intention*, we are not humans having a spiritual experience on earth; we are spiritual beings having a human experience on earth. Teach your daughter the beauty in life and guide her in ways to express herself.

> *Years ago I worked at a cancer center in Lubbock, Texas. I had the good fortune of meeting a splendid young girl there named "Maggie." Maggie was dying of a rare lung cancer. Although she knew it, she never let it slow her down. She played the clarinet, was involved in a jazz band, and had developed an interest in designing clothes. Maggie became so ill with the cancer that she no longer had the lung capacity to blow on the clarinet. What amazed me was she never talked about her bald head or her belly bloat caused by the chemo and steroids. She kept focusing on what she did well. She would bring a sketch book to the hospital and make sketches of new outfits for fall or spring, depending on the season. I told her mother how amazed I was and what a great job she had done to keep her daughter's passion alive, even while she was so sick.*
>
> *Her mother told me that she purposely had raised her daughters to contribute to society. Whatever their dreams were, she introduced avenues so they could explore them. She told me that Maggie had always loved music as a child. Mom took her to concerts, and bands of all types. She had bought Maggie music so*

she could listen to it at bedtime. Maggie became more excited with her music because her mom was excited and interested in it. When Maggie started making drawings of clothes, her mom took her to department stores to look at all the latest fashions. This was a free activity, but it took a lot of time. Mom was smart. She knew she was lighting a fire for Maggie's interests. She didn't ask the babysitter or nanny to take her. She spent the time with her whenever she could, which wasn't easy as a single mother with two children.

Maggie ended up dying, but her mom continues to write to me. She tells me all the time how proud she was of Maggie and how much Maggie had enriched her life. As for me, I have a whole tablet full of Maggie's drawings. She had a passion that continues to live on whenever I look at it, remembering her excitement for something she did that was so very well done.

Some people go to temples, some to churches and still others to synagogues. It doesn't matter where you go, what is important is you respect it, and you make a place for it in your busy lives. Your daughter is watching you all the time. She sees when you go to church and then criticize other people as soon as you drive away. She also sees when you are gracious and display genuine gratitude. You are helping build a foundation with her. Don't ever think she doesn't see you or know what you are doing. She may act like she is preoccupied with her own life and doesn't care about yours. She does care. She also wants you to care and to share her life.

I have always been intrigued why boys grow up so much more confident of what they want to be than our daughters. It is as if the girl puts her own aspirations on hold until she meets a boy or marries, and then supports his career goals instead of her own. I believe some of this occurs because we teach our daughters that they should care for others' needs first—that's the definition of womanhood that they learn. Consequently, they never are sufficiently centered enough that they can find out what their gifts are or their passions.

Q: So what kinds of things can I do to excite my daughter and help her define her passion?

A: Start early. Talk to her. See what her interests are. Do not over-schedule her. Let her have time to think. The following thoughts are for both mom and daughter to sit down together and discuss how you both feel. Let the goal be total understanding of each other, not persuasion of one another. To find your passions—those things that spark you both:

- ❑ Plan at least one hour a week to sit with her or go window shopping.

- ❑ Have sketch pads and journals placed all over the house.

- ❑ Keep brilliant colored markers, pencils, books on every subject around the house.

- ❑ If you watch TV, watch it together. Make TV dates so you can talk about what you watch.

- ❑ Exercise, whether it is walking together or doing a program together. When you work out together, you don't have to talk about the importance of diet and exercise. You are mentoring it.

- ❑ Go to museums, art galleries, bookstores. Take classes. Start early so they also see you as interested in learning.

- ❑ When you see even one interest of your daughter's, get excited. Expose her to all sides of it. Don't claim it as your own. Let her own it, but show her you think it is neat that she enjoys it.

- ❑ Leave books and magazines on tables, open to strategic pages that would attract attention.

Don't ever try to talk your daughter out of a passion. Every creative person who has ever excelled at anything started out at a level that did not look too impressive. Girls need to dream, and they need to know that their dreams are important to their parents.

Q: My daughter recently told me she wants to explore other faiths. She feels like the Catholic faith is not what she believes in. Help! I come from a family of Catholics. Am I losing my daughter?

A: Congratulations! You have raised a daughter who is seeking her own relationship with God. She is telling you in her own way that she wants to feel closer to God, even if she doesn't think the beliefs in which she has been raised hold the answer for her right now. This is a very healthy sign. Your daughter is saying "I want more. I want to feel God more in my life; I want to have my own relationship with God." Your daughter is telling you she is growing up and is starting to think about her own spiritual growth, not just what has been handed down to her.

Do not panic. Instead, try your best to embrace her new journey. Ask her more about what she is looking for in God. What does she believe God is? How does she want to be involved in church? What is her current faith doing for her? What is her current faith lacking? These questions will help her decide what she is missing. Make these questions part of your *family meetings.*

I can tell you from personal experience that I made a big mistake in this area. I missed an important opportunity with my own daughters in exploring their faith because, like you, I feared them leaving *my church*. I did not see the big picture. What happened is they stayed in *my church* until they finished high school. Once they were in college they didn't go to any church. Slowly they (the oldest one; the youngest one is still confused) are discovering who they are with God and where they see themselves in relationship to Him. I am fortunate they still believe in God and have a strong spirituality. Many girls who are pushed or mandated to attend church later quit all together. She may even be telling you that she is questioning faith itself.

Never force your children to believe what you do. It is wiser to start a dialogue and talk with them about what they believe. If it is a family rule that you all go to church together, that is fine, but never make your child feel that they are being punished for what they believe. Her struggle actually means she is seeking, and that is what we all really want for our children. If you seek God, you are looking for God; you have a place for Him.

Understanding and trying to support each other is of supreme importance. If you gave your daughter a solid foundation, she will find her way. Neither of my daughters may end up being Catholic. But I am convinced they will both be very spiritual and have God in their life.

Q: Earlier you mentioned "family meetings." Can you say more about that, especially in developing passion in my girls?

A: I'm glad to talk about the importance of *family meetings*. I believe strongly in them. The family meeting is an opportunity for the family to become a team, everyone feeling value and worth in their opinion. It can be a time of prayer as it was in my family, or it can be done at the table during dinner, or it can be done after dinner when everyone is relaxed. It's important, however, to make it fun. The family meetings are an outgrowth of the mother-daughter table talks we've been suggesting.

Here are possible ideas for family meetings. Try to present them in a manner that is "fun and empowering" for your daughters, letting the conversation flow freely. Talk about how spirituality can be a powerful force in your life.

Start by establishing a day of the week. This can be done via e-mail, with Post-It® notes on back doors or your daughter's mirror. You can put a slip of paper in her lunch bag or gym bag along with her favorite candy, reminding her of when it will be and at what time. You can have her make suggestions also. The meetings do not need to be held at home, although if there is more then one child at home it may be easier.

The rules are set up by the family. You can make them "girls only" or you can include dad. You can make it so anyone talking has to hold the "talking stick" — a favorite wand, stick, or anything special. Or they can be loose, where you say the only rule is everyone must say something to contribute.

The family meeting can be held every week just to talk. Or it can be called by any family member when who feels unheard. You decide. Keep them light, but meaningful. You can use them to plan vacations, or who should do the laundry. The list is endless.

Remember: the reason for the family meeting is to communicate. Each person is respected, all ideas are heard and people's time is valued. The family meeting should be a positive experience in your family.

Q: *Do our table talk conversations always have to be at the table?*

A. The table is a metaphor. It is best if you think of the table as symbolic for making a date with your daughter/mom to come together and talk. Be open, be honest. Play together. We did this naturally when our daughters were small. Why did we stop? We want them to be as great as we always knew they could be. Daughters, your moms need you to reassure them that you do still love them and need their guidance. Nothing gets better if you are both reacting to each other due to stressors. Take time, sit down at the table — wherever you are — and listen.

Don't ask what the world needs.
Ask what makes you come alive,
and go do it.

-Howard Thurman

FINAL THOUGHTS

We've discussed some very important issues in this book from menstruation and routine health care, to birth control, STD's, and body image. Our overall goal is to inspire open communication between mothers and daughters — to generate memorable conversations and unforgettable table talks. We have provided tips for setting the metaphorical table, suggested ideas on what to bring to the table, given examples of how moms and daughters might carry on such "talks-at-the-table." It is our hope to spark dialog about health, sex or whatever; to pique your curiosity with information that even "she" doesn't know, whether that "she" is your mother or your daughter. With conversations that are lighthearted but not lightweight, we hope to see you (mothers and daughters) discussing important, real issues.

Keep in mind, health care providers often see young women after problems occur – problems that might have been avoided if the adolescents had received adequate education, or if they had found opportunities to engage a trusted, meaningful person with their questions. When we mothers fall short in educating our girls about health, sex, and self-esteem, we miss out on our opportunities to prevent potential problems. We cannot count on the schools, our daughters' peers or the mass media to provide our adolescent girls with the information that they need to protect themselves.

Mothers, use this book to aid you to set the table for in-depth conversations with your daughter. Though these issues are not easily discussed between mother and daughter, it is important to have the conversations to ensure her future health and happiness. To educate is to communicate; to communicate is to listen, to ask questions and to share.

Daughters, here we've given you answers to difficult questions. Do you have any more? Think about it. Highlight some questions you'd like more information about. Talk to your mother. These issues are just a part of life.

And remember, "knowledge is power," and once you have the power, use it.

A woman is the full circle.
Within her is the power to
create, nurture, and transform.

-Diane Mariechild

NOTES

INTRODUCTION

(Pg. 13, *school programs*). The notion of providing sex education programs in public schools has been hotly debated, especially regarding *content* and *format* of such programs. If you want to delve further into this issue, a good place to start is Social Security Administration, Maternal and Child Health Services, Separate Program for Abstinence Education, Section 510 (42 U.S.C. 710).

(Pg. 13, *school programs*). For more on current teenage pregnancy rates, see Darrock J.E., Singh S, Frost, J.J., "Differences in teenage pregnancy rates among 5 developed countries: The role of sexual activity and contraceptive use." *Family Planning Perspectives*, 2002, 34-56, as well as Finer, L.B., *Trends in premarital sex in the United States*, 1954-2003, Public Health Reports, Jan-Feb 2007 vol 122 73-78.

(Pg. 14, *mass media*) For a review of how network television has become sexualized, see Kienkel, D. Cope, K. M., Colvin, *Sexual messages on family hour television*: Keiser Family Foundation, 1996.

CHAPTER 1

(Pg. 28, *cramps*) Although rather technical, a good write up on the pervasive impact of cramps for girls and women is, French, L., *Dysmenorrhea*, **American Family Physician,** January 15, 2005 volume 71, number 2.

CHAPTER 6

(Pg. 146, *Body Mass Index*). For more information on computing Body Mass Index (BMI), visit the U.S. Department of Health & Human Services - National Institutes of Health web site at: http://www.nhlbisupport.com/bmi/.

(Pg. 155, *cyberbullying*). For more on helping your child develop safe internet practices, check out WiredSafety's site: www.wiredsafety.org, It provides help, information and education to Internet and mobile device users of all ages. They help victims of cyberabuse ranging from online fraud, cyberstalking and child safety, to hacking and malicious code attacks. They also help parents with issues, such as MySpace and cyberbullying.

Not everything that is faced can be changed, but nothing can be changed until it is faced.

—James Baldwin

GLOSSARY

A brief guide to unusual terms, medical terms, or common terms used by teens.

Amenorrhea is the absence of your menstrual cycle. Primary amenorrhea means you have never had a period; secondary amenorrhea means you have previously had at least one cycle.

Bacterial Vaginosis is a common vaginal infection caused by an imbalance of normal bacterial growth in the vagina.

Candidiasis is another word for yeast infection caused by an overgrowth of Candida; a common form of vaginal infection.

Chlamydia is a sexually transmitted infection that, if untreated, can cause scarring in tubes and ovaries leading to infertility.

Corpus Luteum is what is left behind in the ovary after ovulation, and it produces progesterone.

Dysmenorrhea refers to menstrual cramps, painful periods.

Endometriosis is a condition where tissue from the lining of the uterus gets misplaced anywhere in the pelvis outside of the uterus including the ovaries and fallopian tubes; a common source of pelvic pain.

Endometrium is the lining of the uterus.

Estrogen is a female hormone produced by the ovaries that causes the lining of the uterus to thicken up most prominent during the beginning of your cycle.

Follicle is a small fluid filled sac that forms in the ovaries that can produce an egg.

Gonorrhea is a sexually transmitted infection that can cause infertility, pelvic inflammatory disease and arthritis if untreated.

Hormones are substances produced by the body that travel through the bloodstream to control certain organs. Estrogen and progesterone are examples of female hormones.

Hirsutism is excessive hair growth on the face chest or abdomen in women, often due to overproduction of testosterone.

Human Papilloma Virus (HPV) is a very common viral infection spread through sexual contact. It is the common virus associated with abnormal Pap tests and cervical cancer.

Mastodynia means painful breasts.

Pap test is a test that looks at cells from the uterine cervix, useful in detecting cervical cancer.

Books

Blackstone, Margaret and Guest, Elissa Haden. (2006) *Girl Stuff: A Survival Guide to Growing Up*. New York: Harcourt. *Another girl-friendly book, exploring both the physical and psychological aspects of puberty. Definitely for girls, not for moms, but it puts important topics on the table in simple, inviting ways.*

Boteach, Shmuley. (2006) *Ten Conversations You Need to Have with Your Children*. New York, NY: HarperCollins. *Though not as focused on sexuality and personal health as our book, we find Boteach's approach to be an excellent foundation.*

Canfield, Jack and Victor-Hansen, Mark. (2007) *Life Lessons for Busy Moms: Essential Ingredients to Organize and Balance Your Work*. Deerfield Beach, FL: Health Communications, Inc. *Among other things, these Chicken Soup for the Soul® authors remind us not to forget our children in our busy lives.*

Canfield, Jack; Victor-Hansen, Mark; Hansen, Patty; and Dunlap, Irene. (2005) *Chicken Soup for the Girl's Soul*. Deerfield Beach, FL: Health Communications, Inc. *In traditional Chicken Soup for the Soul® style, real stories by real girls about real stuff. The short excerpts serve as excellent mother-daughter conversation starters.*

Clifford-Poston, Andrea. (2005) *Tweens: Understanding Your 8-12 Year Old*. Oxford, England: Oneworld Publications. *Solid, readable, practical; not overly psychological.*

Cline, Foster W. and Fay, Jim. (2006) *Parenting Teens With Love And Logic*. Deerfield Beach, FL: Pinon Press. *This therapeutic approach originally designed for children with attachment disorders provides invaluable advice for dealing with daughters of all ages and temperaments.*

Cohen-Sandler, Roni. (2005) *Stressed Out Girls*. New York, NY: Penguin.
A good book, but it focuses on the abnormal psyche of girls and
what happens when girls go bad.

Elium, Jeanne and Elium, Don. (2003) *Raising a Daughter: Parents and the
Awakening of a Healthy Woman*. Berkeley, CA: Ten Speed Press.
Practical exploration of what it means to have a daughter, and how
cultural forces impact becoming a woman today. For those moms
interested in "the bigger picture."

Eyre, Linda and Eyre, Richard. (1999) *How to Talk to Your Child about
Sex*. New York, NY: Martin's Press.
The Eyres' book is almost ten years old now, but the advice is
every bit up-to-date.

Devillers, Julia. (2002) *GirlWise: How to Be Confident, Capable, Cool and
in Control*. New York, NY: Three Rivers Press.
Not really about body development nor about sexuality, but
definitely a girl-friendly book written after our own heart. Great
read!

Drill, Esther and McDonald, Heather. (1999) *Deal with It! A Whole New
Approach to Your Body, Brain and Life as a gURL*.
A girl-friendly, hilarious, yet "deep" book for girls from gURL.com,
the largest community of teenage girls on the web. The whole book
matches the look and feel of the web site; definitely in sync with
today's teen. We especially like their straightforward focus on self-
responsibility.

Fleming, Don. (1993) *How to Stop the Battle with Your Teenager*. New
York, NY: Fireside.
For both boys and girls; helpful in a very practical way to guide
you through everyday land mines. Focuses on accepting that our
children do have problems—accept it, don't get defensive about
it. We use it in our clinical practices as a wonderful resource with
practical applications.

Gabriel, H. Paul, M.D., and Wool ,Robert. (1995) *Anticipating
Adolescence*. New York: Henry Holt and Company.
Describes ways to deal with specific problems during the
unpredictable teen years, keeping relationships intact.

Ginsburg, K.R. (2002) *"But I'm Almost 13."* Chicago, IL: Contemporary
Press.
A book for parents to improve communication between mothers

*and teens. We like this book because there are some very useful
tips on how to effectively communicate with adolescents.*

Jackson, Nisha. (2006). *Surviving the Teenage Hormone Takeover (A
    Guide for Moms).* New York, NY: Thomas Nelson.
    *This book goes through common problems that girls experience
    on their way to adulthood. The basic premise is that girls need
    their moms to help them on this journey. After each problem is
    discussed, suggestions are offered on how you as a mom can help.
    Although you may not find the suggestions earth shaking, it will be
    more of a gentle reminder that you are needed, and may give you
    ideas on what you may do to help your daughter at that time. It is
    beneficial mostly to raise awareness.*

Madaras, Lynda and Madaras, Area. (2000) *My Body, My Self: For Girls.*
    New York, NY: Newmarket Press.
    *A perennial bestselling classic for preteen girls. An excellent
    starting place for some of the basics about body development.*

Marshner, Connie. (1988) *Decent Exposure: How to Teach Your Children
    about Sex.* Nashville, TN: Wolgemuth & Hyatt Pub.
    *We listed this book because it is a detailed philosophical book
    about teaching morality, religion and sexuality—essentially putting
    "God back into sex." This book would work well in private
    schools with religious doctrines, but is also a good conversation
    starter for any mom and daughter.*

McCarthy, Moira. (2008) *The Everything Guide to Raising Adolescent
    Girls.* Avon, MA: Adams Media.
    *Part of the Adams Media "The Everything Series," which are
    designed to be handy, accessible books tackling difficult topics.
    Definitely for moms, not for daughters, it gives you a smattering
    of lots of good topics, including how to talk about sex, dating and
    "risky business" on the internet. An easy skim.*

McMahon, Tom. (2003) *Teen Tips: A Practical Survival Guide for Parents
    with Kids 11 to 19.* New York, NY: Pocket.
    *A wonderful light-hearted guide for everything kid-related. It is
    best used as a resource along side other books that address more
    serious problems. It deals with sleep-overs as well as curfews. You
    will be hard pressed to find a topic it doesn't address; however the
    advice is limited and brief. We like it as a quick referral, and we
    enjoy the lightness of the book.*

Meeker, Meg. (2007) *Your Kids at Risk: How Teen Sex Threatens Our Sons and Daughters*. Washington, DC: Regency Publishing.
Well researched and thought-provoking; you're sure to have some conversations with your daughter after working your way through this book.

Northrup, Christiane. (2005). *Mother-Daughter Wisdom: Understanding the Crucial Link between Mothers, Daughters, and Health*. New York, NY: Bantam Dell.
Dr. Northrup, bestselling author and trusted, visionary medical expert, provides a blueprint for women of all ages to understand health, relationships and feminine power. Exceptional resource.

Richardson, Justin and Schuster, Mark. (2003) *Everything You Never Wanted Your Kids to Know about Sex (But Were Afraid They'd Ask): The Secrets to Surviving Your Child's Sexual Development from Birth to the Teens*. New York, NY: Three Rivers Press.
An excellent, up-to-date compilation of research and interviews. Done with wit and wisdom. Though not specific to teenage girls, a handy book for those unexpected questions.

Riera, Michael. (2003) *Staying Connected to Your Teenager: How to Keep Them Talking to You and How to Hear What They're Really Saying*. Cambridge, MA: Da Capo Press.
A handy guide for conversations in general. We like the focus on connection.

Schafer, Ayson. (2006) *Breaking the Good Mom Myth*. Somerset, NJ: John Wiley & Sons.
Like the rest of Wiley books, great for moms and for therapists.

Shalit, Wendy. (2007) *Girls Gone Mild: Young Women Reclaim Self-Respect and Find It's Not Bad to Be Good*. New York, NY: Random House.
A little different slant, but it might spark some conversations between moms and daughters, especially when comparing it to our book.

Shearin Karres, Erika V. (2004) *Mean Chicks, Cliques, and Dirty Tricks*. Avon, MA: Adams Media Corporation / F+W Publications.
Like the title suggests, straightforward advice on girl teenage relationships.

Synderman, Nancy and Streep, Peg. (2002) *Girl in the Mirror: Mothers and Daughters in the Years of Adolescence*. New York, NY: Hyperion. *Like Elium's book, a joyful read on the philosophical, cultural, and psychological issues of emerging womanhood. We especially appreciate the focus on teenage years as an opportunity to celebrate —rather than simply "survive"— the mother-daughter connection.*

van Munching, Philip. (2005) *Boys Will Put You on a Pedestal (So They Can Look Up Your Skirt): A Dad's Advice for Daughters*. New York, NY: Simon & Schuster. *In writing this touching, funny love letter to his daughters, van Munching has given each of us a valuable blueprint for broaching some of life's touchy issues with our children. More an inspirational read than a guide, it fits very well with our focus on parent-daughter conversations.*

Wiseman, Rosalind. (2003) *Queen Bees and Wanna Bees*. London, England: Piatkus Books. *Anyone who has a daughter should read this book. It is written in a way that makes you laugh as well as cry. You will find yourself asking "Is my daughter a Queen Bee or a wanna be?" By the end you will be trying to place yourself in one of the categories as well. If you never understood the stress your daughter feels among her peers, you will after reading this book.*

ORGANIZATIONS, WEB SITES, AND HOT LINES

Digene HPVTest
<http://www.theHPVTest.com>
We love Digene Corporations's web site because it gives straight-forward, factual information about HPV as well as treatment.

Centers for Disease Control and Prevention (Department of Health and Human Resources)
<http://www.cdc.gov/STD>
This is an excellent web site to obtain facts concerning sexually transmitted infections.

CDC Sexually Transmitted Diseases Hot Line
800-227-8922

National Eating Disorder Association
800-931-2237

Families Are Talking (part of The Family Project of the Sexuality
Information and Education Council of the United States [SIECUS]).
<http://www.familiesaretalking.org>
*This project began in 2000 to empower parents and caregivers to
communicate with their children about sexuality-related issues. We
send families to this site because it tackles most of the problems
families bring to therapy. It addresses boundary issues, issues with
friends, how to start a family budget. It also is a parent-friendly
source: very direct and easy to access.*

American Social Health Association (ASHA)
<http://www.iwannaknow.org>
<http://www.ashastd.org>
*ASHA runs the www.iwannaknow.org[SM] web sites, which is one
of the best sites for teens to read about sexuality and relationships.
It has reliable, up-to-date information on birth control and also
addresses relationship problems that are common for the teenage
population.*

teenwire.com of the Planned Parenthood Federation of America (PPFA)
<http://www.teenwire.com>
*An award-winning sexual health web site for teens, teenwire.com
offers bilingual (English/Spanish) information on sexuality as well
as healthy living for teens. It provides in-depth reference articles as
well as links to other sites to explore. It is wonderful because of its
ethnic diversity.*

Something Fishy
<http://www.somethingfishy.org>
*We believe this is one of the best sites for eating disorders. We use
it in the Weight Management Center. It is not focused on food but
rather on the compulsions as well as addictions that manifest as
eating disorder. This site is helpful for parents, teens, as well as
professionals.*

BodyPositive®
<http://www.bodypositive.com>
*This is an excellent site to be used in conjunction with family
meetings or "date nights" with your teenage daughter. It has
meditations, mindful eating activities, exercises, as well as articles
about accepting your body. It leaves you feeling empowered which
is why it is one of our favorite sites.*

INDEX

ABOUT THE AUTHORS

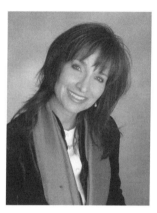

Mary Jo Rapini, M.Ed., LPC is featured on TLC's new series, *Big Medicine*. She is an intimacy and sex counselor, certified anger management therapist, and popular speaker. A mom with two daughters, her passion is helping all girls become strong women.

Janine J. Sherman, RN-C, MSN is a women's health care nurse practitioner. Both her patients and her two daughters come to her for answers to their biggest questions about health and sexuality. Now you can, too.

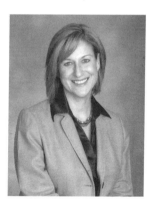

Please visit Mary Jo and Janine at www.StartTalkingBook.com.

ORDERING INFORMATION

Additional copies of *Start Talking: A Girl's Guide for You and Your Mom about Health, Sex, or Whatever* from the publisher. Orders may be placed by phone, by mail, by FAX, or directly on the web. Purchase orders from institutions are welcome.

❏ *To order by mail:* Complete this order form and mail it (along with check or credit card information) to Bayou Publishing, 2524 Nottingham, Houston, TX 77005-1412.

❏ *To order by phone:* Call (800) 340-2034.

❏ *To order by FAX:* Fill out this order form (including credit card information) and fax to (713) 526-4342.

❏ *To place a secure online order:* Visit http://www.bayoupublishing.com.

Name: _____

Address: _____

_____

City: _____ ST: ___ Zip: _____

Ph: _____

FAX: _____

E-mail: _____

❏ VISA ❏ MasterCard ❏ American Express ❏ Discover

Charge Card #: _____

Expiration Date: _____

Signature: _____

Please send me _____ copies at $14.95 each _____

Sales Tax 8.25%(Texas residents) _____

plus $4.50 postage and handling *(per order)* _____$4.50

Total $ _____

Bayou Publishing
2524 Nottingham, Suite 150
Houston, TX 77005-1412
Ph: (713) 526-4558/ FAX: (713) 526-4342
Orders: (800) 340-2034
http://www.bayoupublishing.com